LABOR OF LOVE

Labor of Love

Mothers Share the Joy of Childbirth

Judith Zimmer

John Wiley & Sons, Inc.
New York • Chichester • Weinheim • Toronto • Singapore • Brisbane

Copyright © 1997 by Judith Zimmer
Published by John Wiley & Sons, Inc.

Library of Congress Cataloging-in-Publication Data

Zimmer, Judith.
    Labor of love: mothers share the joy of childbirth / Judith Zimmer.
        p.   cm.
    Includes bibliographical references and index.
    ISBN 0-471-15703-1 (pbk.: alk. paper)
    1. Childbirth—Case studies.   2. Labor (Obstetrics)—Case studies.
  I. Title.
  RG652.Z54   1997
  618.4—dc20   96-35910

Printed in the United States of America

10 9 8 7 6 5 4 3 2 1

This book is for all expectant mothers,
with the hope that they too will have positive
childbirth experiences.

CONTENTS

Contents

FOREWORD

It has been almost thirty years since I gave birth to my first child. My memories of labor and delivery are vague, partially because I had a fair amount of sedation which was common in 1967. Yet having a new baby was the most incredible thing I had ever experienced. I wanted to capture the joy and wonder of the birth of my firstborn, Wendy, so the day after she was born, I felt compelled to write down some of my thoughts and feelings. Rereading it today, I realize how little control I had over the actual birth process.

My second and third babies were premature and so no anesthesia could be administered. My pain during each of those experiences was heightened by fear for the baby.

Because I was older than many of my friends when they had their children, I don't remember comparing birthing stories. However, everyone I knew had their babies in a hospital. In the late sixties and early seventies women weren't allowed to make many decisions regarding labor and delivery; most of us didn't question that practice.

Now my twenty-nine-year-old daughter is pregnant with her first child and I see a world of difference. She is asking many more questions. I'm happy that I am able to provide her with some information because I've been involved with research on pregnancy ever since 1982, when I cofounded Melpomene Institute for Women's Health Research.

Melpomene Institute was created to fill the gap in knowledge about the link between physical activity and women's health. We conduct research projects that are practical in nature.

One of our most important goals is to make our findings available to women so they can make their own informed decisions.

One of our first projects was to look at the relationship between exercise and pregnancy. Many women had been physically active, some at a competitive level, before becoming pregnant. These women wanted to remain active but they didn't want to harm their growing babies. Many were unhappy with their physicians' lack of knowledge on the subject. The common medical stance was to be fairly cautious, telling pregnant women to restrict their exercise drastically.

Melpomene research found that physical activity is not only safe for most pregnant women, but that it enhances pregnancy. A main benefit of exercise during pregnancy is psychological. One woman wrote, "Exercise gives me an alive feeling. Pregnancy is a natural state; you are limited, but by no means incapable. My spirits soared as I walked and dreamed and talked to our baby. You get more oxygen and so does the baby. Inactivity causes a vicious cycle of fatigue."

Women also told us that being physically active helped them accept their changing body and shape. "At first my body image and self-esteem suffered," said one woman, "I've always been thin and it was hard to feel that I looked fat. I felt out of control. Going swimming several times a week made me appreciate the sleekness of my body. I realized fat related to pregnancy was healthy."

Many women hoped that physical activity during pregnancy would guarantee a short labor. Our studies did not find any relationship between fitness and length of labor, but many women told us that being athletic helped them cope with labor. In fact, many women told us that labor was more difficult than any physical feat they had accomplished. Many also told us there were many similarities between childbirth and running a marathon or completing some other major physical challenge. "I've experienced pain as an athlete," said one woman,

"I visualized the end of labor as I had previously visualized the end of the triathlon. It made it seem much easier."

Being aware of what was happening to their bodies gave the women in the Melpomene studies a sense that they could make the changes and adaptations necessary to achieve the best possible outcome for their babies and themselves.

We did a second study on exercise and pregnancy that began in 1983, and we have remained interested in the pregnancy experience ever since. At first we were amazed that Melpomene's information on exercise and pregnancy would remain one of our most popular topics over the years, but good information on the role of physical activity is still hard to find.

Clearly women have begun to take a more active role in their pregnancies in the last decade. While there are many more books available on a wide range of pregnancy topics, I had not found anything I could highly recommend about the birth process itself until I read this book.

Labor of Love: Mothers Share the Joy of Childbirth is a compilation of stories that reflect the wide range of choices available to women. The stories are a fast and interesting read, yet full of factual medical advice that I have not seen elsewhere.

Judith Zimmer tells us that she became interested in positive childbirth stories because of her personal experience. Her own labor and delivery was much longer than anticipated, yet she found the experience very joyful and uplifting. Listening to other women, however, she found that horror stories were related more often than positive ones. She began looking for other women who felt as she did. As she listened to other women who enjoyed their births, she found that while some had natural childbirth and others had C-sections, epidurals, or VBACs, they all took the time to choose the kind of birth that was right for them. They selected their practitioners with great care, asking lots of questions as well as going with the flow of events during labor. It is the diversity of their experiences and the different ways they dealt with change that make this book so useful.

You may want to read all 19 stories at once or to read a few at a time. The fact that there are so many different options enables you to read more closely about the option your hope and expect will transpire. I recommend that you at least skim most of them, because you never can predict exactly what your own experience will be. You'll see that no matter what happens, it's important that you participate in the decision-making process. It's also important to be flexible enough to change course as the situation demands. The bottom line is that a healthy baby is the most important thing.

One of the aspects I particularly like about this book is that helpful facts are interspersed throughout the stories. For example, one of the women describes her experience with pre-eclampsia, and Zimmer adds a paragraph that explains, in understandable medical terms, what was going on and how common the problem is.

Judith Zimmer is an excellent writer and I hope and believe that this book will help expectant mothers think through their choices. I recommend you use the practical advice offered in the book's final section as you consider your own birth options.

I'm excited to have this book to add to the Melpomene Institute's resources for women. It fits perfectly with our philosophy that an educated woman provides herself with the best choices for a healthy lifestyle. By sharing stories and good practical advice, Judith Zimmer helps you prepare for your own positive birthing experience.

Judy Mahle Lutter
President, Melpomene Institute for Women's Health Research

ACKNOWLEDGMENTS

I would like to thank the 18 women who so eagerly shared their birth stories with me—Joanna Allen, Ann Arscott, Miriam Block, Susan Bjornson, Annette Cantor, Barbara Cattermole, Beth Curry, Kari Garcia Fisher, Liz Benson Forer, Jane Gerson, Val Harper, Megan Howard, Rosemary Moore, Susan Olman, Vicki Placha, Ivy Ratafia, Tal Recanati, and Sarah Ryan. I appreciate the time they gave and their willingness to be part of this collection. This book is theirs.

Many thanks also to Samantha McCormick, midwife-to-be, of ICAN/NYC, who e-mailed answers to my questions with speed and grace, to Lois Metzger for reading early drafts, to Janina Quint for helping me find terrific women to interview, and to Danielle Mailer for being part of this book. Thank you to Angela Miller for encouraging me, and to Judith McCarthy for believing in this book from the beginning. A final note of thanks to Barbara Sellars and Carol Bronte of CBS Midwifery in New York City, who helped me define positive childbirth. And especially to Barbara who was with me the day I lived the idea of this book—October 4, 1991, the day Sam was born.

INTRODUCTION

Positive. It's a word rarely used in connection with childbirth. Yet this book shares the stories of women who speak in glowing terms of the joy of giving birth. They're not talking about seeing or holding the baby for the first time, but the actual birth process. This isn't to say that labor was necessarily short or that it wasn't painful. Regardless of the way they gave birth—naturally, with drugs, or with other medical interventions—these women say they had some control over their bodies and the process of giving birth. They didn't blindly hand themselves over to a doctor or to technology. Instead, they accepted the challenges of childbirth by realizing the importance of the birth experience to themselves and to their unborn child, by being actively involved in the birthing process and the decisions surrounding it, and by trusting themselves and their bodies.

"Having a positive birth experience is empowering," explains Barbara Sellars, a certified nurse-midwife in New York City. "It makes you feel as though you can accomplish great things. What better way is there to start off as a parent?"

Unfortunately, many of us hear childbirth horror stories more frequently than positive birthing stories. Although there is no qualitative research to date on childbirth satisfaction, I have been conducting my own informal survey and have found that you actually have to seek out positive stories—they don't just come flooding at you.

Let me explain: I became interested in positive childbirth experiences because I almost didn't have one. I had a slow, two-day labor and gave birth to a baby whose size—9 pounds 11 ounces—shocked everyone. Because of the length of my labor and the size of my baby, I probably would have been a candidate for cesarean section (C-section) if I hadn't switched from a high-tech obstetrician to a midwife in my seventh month. Instead, I experienced a very fulfilling birth in the manner and setting I chose.

After becoming a mother, I began listening to other women's childbirth experiences with an ear toward hearing other positive stories. I could always tell when I'd found a kindred soul by a certain heightened pleasure and assured tone in the voice. The women I talked to didn't all have natural (unmedicated), vaginal deliveries. Some had epidurals, others VBACs, and still others C-sections. I realized that, no matter how we had delivered, we had certain traits in common. We'd done our homework beforehand; we'd chosen our practitioners with great care and asked lots of questions. We'd also gone with the flow of events, the subtle changes and little (or big) surprises that labor can bring. We'd participated in the decision-making process (as much as possible). We'd changed course as necessary. And we realized that a healthy baby was more important than the birth itself.

It was disconcerting for me to find that such positive childbirth stories were few and far between and that it wasn't common to find women who loved their birth experience.

When you consider what happens during a lot of births, it isn't any wonder that more women aren't reporting a more satisfactory experience. There are several choices about where to deliver and with whom, but most women decide to have a doctor deliver their baby in a hospital. (My guess is that many women think this is the only choice available to them—and, of course, for some it is.) In many hospitals, and with most doctors, the usual procedure is to use drugs, including painkillers or anesthesia. Intervention techniques, such as IVs and electronic fetal monitoring (which are known to slow down labor and make a woman immobile), have become so commonplace that they are often considered standard practice. Once the chain of drugs and intervention starts, more complications tend to occur. The United States boasts the highest C-section rate in the world, peaking at 24.7 percent of all births in 1988 and decreasing to 21.8 percent in 1993.

With such widespread intervention and so many C-sections, is it any wonder that one of the most often-heard complaints from women is that, through the course of labor and delivery at a hospital with a physician, the medical team takes over and the mother loses control of her baby's birth? And is it any wonder that, because of the current state of birth in America, many women face labor and delivery with fear rather than with the attitude that their body is meant to do this?

The myths and stories surrounding childbirth reinforce the idea that women are meant to suffer in childbirth. The Genesis story of Eve is a prime example. God curses Eve for her sins by saying, "In sorrow shalt thou bring forth children." The pain she will suffer in childbirth is inevitable. Do we continue to live out Eve's punishment even today?

Through the ages, writers have told us that the pain of labor is one of the worst in human life. Often the way cultures react to this expected pain tells us a lot about them. In some cultures, it is traditional not to utter a word when in pain; in others, people scream their way through labor and delivery. Take the childbirth scenes in literature. In *War and Peace*, for example, Princess Lise makes "piteous, helpless, animal moans" during childbirth. At one point, her husband looks at her in labor and thinks her eyes seem to say, "I have done no one any harm: Why must I suffer like this? Help me!" A description like this (the creation of a man) makes it seem as though all women in labor are beyond help.

It seems clear that we don't expect much from ourselves. Because of our baggage surrounding this event, it comes as no surprise that prospective parents face childbirth with dread and fear. But it doesn't have to be that way.

It isn't that there is no pain during childbirth—there usually is. And no one should expect otherwise. But it is pain with a purpose. And knowing that can change everything—including your outlook toward the pain. Labor can be difficult and intense, but along with the pain comes the joy of one of the most amazing moments a woman can experience—the birth of her child.

Women face other challenges in their lives (running marathons, for example) by not focusing on the pain but by welcoming the challenge—to see if they can do it or how far they can go. As Adrienne Rich writes in *Of Woman Born*, "Rarely has [childbirth] been viewed as one way of knowing and coming to terms with our bodies, of discovering our physical and psychic resources."

It's important to remember that childbirth is not an isolated event in a woman's or a couple's life. The choices we make about where we deliver and with whom reflect our feelings about ourselves and our bodies. These choices affect our unborn baby—from the drugs we take (which can affect the baby's neurological system both short- and long-term) to the amount of time a hospital allows the mother and her baby to spend together immediately after birth.

The way we handle ourselves during childbirth is symbolic of the way we live in the world. "The real issue, underlying the economic profit of the medical profession," writes Rich, "is the mother's relation to childbirth, an experience in which women have historically felt out of control, at the mercy of biology, fate, or chance. To change the experience of childbirth means to change women's relationship to fear and powerlessness, to our bodies, to our children; it has far-reaching psychic and political implications."

The collection of birth stories in this book is an attempt to begin that change—to inspire women to find ways of making childbirth better for themselves. These women did. Their stories demonstrate that you can, too, regardless of the manner in which you plan to give birth. *Positiveness*, as it relates to all kinds of childbirth, is an idea whose time has come.

In today's world of childbirth interventions and high C-section rates, the question we need to ask ourselves is how we can make the best use of medical and technological advantages (such as painkillers and electronic fetal monitoring), rather than having them take advantage of us. The birth stories in this book illustrate that you can use painkillers to help you and that, in some cases, a C-section can be the best delivery method for you and your baby. Perhaps we are already approaching the time when women are able to say that there is not just one ideal way of giving birth.

In researching this book, I contacted several women involved in childbirth reform. I explained that I was looking for positive childbirth stories, including C-section stories. One woman just laughed at me. She told me that all C-sections end in tears and that I'd never find positive stories. I hope that I have proved her wrong with the stories included here.

But she was right about one thing. The search wasn't always easy. I selected C-section stories with great care; for example, I chose not to include the story of a woman who wanted a C-section for no other reason than to avoid labor. Instead, I wanted stories that demonstrated a positive way of dealing with the complications of pregnancy and delivery.

One point about C-sections that bears clarification is that there *is* a high C-section rate in this country and that many C-sections aren't necessary. Especially in the VBAC stories, you will see examples of women whose births were taken away from them: Beth Curry's and Ivy Ratafia's first births are described in their VBAC stories. But other stories reveal how C-sections save the lives of both women and their babies. This happened to Sarah Ryan (who tried a home birth), Megan Howard (whose baby was too big for a safe vaginal delivery), Jane Gerson (who had herpes), and Kari Garci Fisher (who had preeclampsia).

With our eyes fixed on the national C-section rate, we often forget these women, belittling all women who have had C-sections. Some tend to do the same thing to women who use painkillers or have epidurals to help them. We deny these women a sense of achievement. I have had friends who were uncomfortable admitting to me that they had an epidural because they assumed that I thought that everyone's birth should be natural like mine. But my feeling is that no woman should be made to feel slighted by her childbirth experience. Sometimes intervention and painkillers can be used as tools for a positive birth. It is wrong to imply that natural childbirth is the only good or right birth. And it seems as though that's the trap that many childbirth reformers have fallen into. (It's interesting to note, however, that practitioners like midwives tend to take a more practical stand. They know, they have seen, that natural childbirth is not for everyone.) I'd like to see us expand our definition of positive childbirth. *What's right for you is what's best for you and your baby.* That's the message you'll get from these birth stories. And, through these stories, I hope that you'll retain a little bit of positiveness for yourself and your own birth. Part Five of this book offers some suggestions to consider as you anticipate your own joyful birth experience.

The great thing about birth stories is that we learn from them. They widen our experience and bring us a little closer to what our own experience might be like. Many women have told me that birth stories were all they wanted to hear and read about before going into labor. The stories here show how similar all births are, and yet how different. I know of no better way to prepare for childbirth than to follow the details of other mothers' stories, especially those who are satisfied with their experience.

These birth stories speak for themselves. Through them, I hope you will learn how to find the joy in your own childbirth experience, to make it your own—something you can be proud of.

My own birth story is part of this collection, and I know that I am in very good company, indeed.

6

PART ONE

Natural Childbirth Stories

🌿 1

Judith's Story

A Last-Minute Change to a Midwife

I was more afraid of the drugs and the IV than of labor. So, late in my pregnancy, I decided to leave the high-tech doctor I'd known for five years and have my baby delivered in a hospital with a midwife.

In my first trimester, I was so absorbed with being pregnant that giving birth seemed far away, like something that was going to happen to someone else. It was a few months before I began to ask my obstetrician questions about the way she delivered babies.

I had always had a good relationship with this doctor. She'd been my gynecologist for five years, and I'd always hoped she would deliver my first child. During each visit to her office, I asked questions of her or of her two female partners as I rotated among the three of them. I told my doctor that I wanted to have as natural a birth as possible. She said that I should keep my options open, that I didn't really know what childbirth was like, so how could I know what I wanted? During each visit, I probed further. What about squatting? She didn't recommend it. Would I be constantly hooked up to a monitor? Yes, the hospital required it.

Like many women, I hadn't even known which hospital my gynecologist was affiliated with. It's not the kind of question you ask when you are just seeing someone for routine Pap smears and checkups. Later, I found out that hers was one of the more high-tech hospitals in the city—great for high-risk pregnancies, which mine was not.

I left each doctor's visit trying to piece together the information I'd heard. I planned my questions carefully and continued to ask them. I always hated the answers I got. I began to worry. Something wasn't right, and I could feel it in my gut. I felt uneasy. I heard about a friend's natural birth with a midwife and was envious. I wanted that kind of birth. "You love your doctor," said my husband. "You'll never leave her."

Would I be able to?

Then came the deciding issue. One day, I asked one of the partners about the use of an IV. If everything was going well—the labor was progressing, and the baby was fine—did you still need one? The answer was yes. The IV would contain either water or sugar water to keep me hydrated (mainly because the hospital didn't allow laboring women to drink or eat). That did it. Having an IV inserted into my arm no matter what (instead of being able to just drink water) was not my idea of a good time. I was more afraid of the IV and how it would make me feel (sick, unwell, bloody) than of the labor itself. I was seven months pregnant. I realized I had to do something.

It turned out that the hospital in my neighborhood worked with several midwives. One midwife group gave a weekly orientation and tour at the hospital. I met all four women in the practice and felt comfortable immediately. In one evening, I found out everything I needed to know about their practice and philosophy. Hearing that their ideas were similar to mine was a relief, and I began to feel as though the person who delivered my baby didn't have to be my best friend, just someone I agreed with. I could feel something settle in me, as though the baby was happy we'd made this change.

10

Telling my doctor I was leaving was more difficult than I thought. She didn't take it well. She called me on the phone and told me that she would deliver my baby the way I wanted, and she'd guarantee that she'd be there. She told me that I would have a better birth experience with her than with anyone else—a sell job. I think she never believed that I'd leave. But I did, spending the next two months rotating among the four midwives.

I tried to slow down my work schedule a week before my due date, which was September 28. But when there was no sign of labor, and I was just waiting around, I did some more work—at home, sitting on the couch, legs up, to be more comfortable. During the days that followed, I took a walk in the morning and had an ongoing conversation with a neighbor about dates and birthdays. I half believed my baby would be born in early October because no one in my family is born at the end of a month. I also thought the birth would occur on an even-numbered day (another family tradition).

The first real sign of labor came late on Tuesday night, October 1, at about 11:30 P.M. It felt like menstrual cramps that were already beyond the normal. I walked around my loft a few times. It was hard to stay still. This lasted for two hours. I started bleeding. I knew bleeding could be part of early labor, but this was more than I'd expected. I telephoned the midwife on call, and she said bleeding was normal. She was in the middle of delivering twins and said, "Don't come in tonight. It's too busy." I obeyed. I had a few more irregular contractions and went to sleep. I realized when I woke up in the morning that I had slept and that the contractions were gone. That morning, I talked to another midwife on call, and she said those contractions didn't count because they'd stopped.

Wednesday, October 2, was another ordinary, wait-for-labor day. I had no real contractions. I did some work, browsed in a bookstore, and sat in the park with a friend and had tea.

11

Another friend walked by and said, "No baby yet?" Not yet. I went to bed that evening and woke up at 1:30 A.M. with *real* contractions. I started timing them, and they were 10 to 15 minutes apart. I didn't feel comfortable lying down, so I spent much of the night on the couch in the living room, looking out the window at a tall building in Chinatown, wondering why so many lights were on in the early morning. What were the people doing up at that hour?

I was a little tired, having been up the night before. I did the exercise I'd been taught in Bradley class, relaxing before a contraction. The problem with sleeping or lying down during a contraction was that I'd fall asleep and then wake up in the middle of it, rather than being ready for it from the beginning. I dozed on and off that night in a sitting position. And I dreamed. Each contraction became a person: an old man, an old woman, a young woman. I could tell whether it was an old man contraction or an old woman. I liked the woman's contractions more than the man's. The man's were more intense and painful. I also remember dreaming that each contraction was a corporation: the McHenry Contraction, the Simmons Contraction—although I don't know where this came from or where it was going.

By the morning, the contractions were 7 to 10 minutes apart and regular. My husband, Alastair, woke up and helped me time them. When I threw up, we both thought this would be the real thing. I called the midwives early that morning, around eight. Barbara was at home. I thought vomiting might mean something: Could it be transition already? She made me talk through a contraction, her way of gauging how tough it was. I think I sounded pretty good. The contractions were painful, but bearable. She said to stay in touch. She'd call from rounds at the hospital. Then the contractions started to slow down again, hovering back around 10 to 15 minutes. No big business here. I wasn't relieved, though, I was really ready to get this show on the road.

We hung out at home all day. Alastair worked on the computer. Every time a contraction started, I'd yell out, "Now," and he'd time it. After a while, we had pages and pages of little green stick'ems with the contraction times written down. I had an appointment with the midwives that afternoon. Instead, Barbara made a house call and came over at about 3 P.M. She examined me and found I was three centimeters dilated.

She wasn't sure whether we'd see her later that day, that night, or the next day. I was in stall mode. She left, and I took a shower. Then things really started. The contractions started coming strong and steady, about four to five minutes apart. I kept hoping they'd continue. They got worse, and the only thing I could do was rock back and forth, standing in front of a low wooden chest in the bedroom. I was happy to be in so much pain because I didn't want to wait any longer or spend another night with mild contractions. It was exciting and not yet serious. Alastair and I timed. We called Barbara while she was still at the office to tell her about the progress. We called her back in another hour to report that things were still going strong. She called the hospital and made arrangements for us to go over there. There was only one labor bed left, and she wanted us to get it; so we left for the hospital around 6 P.M.

We took a cab through Greenwich Village to the hospital. Every time now that I drive on 9th Street, I remember going to the hospital. I was very self-contained and calm during the drive—not at all how I imagined it to be. At the hospital, we found Barbara at the elevators. There was another woman in labor who was on a stretcher. She'd been at the Maternity Center (a birthing center) and was being transferred. Her midwife said, "I have a woman in labor here." Barbara turned to everyone and said, "I do, too." And there I was, standing in the corner of the elevator, quietly handling the contractions.

The room we were shown to wasn't a real birthing room, although I wouldn't have known the difference if Barbara hadn't told us. From the window, we had a great view of the Empire State Building, all lit up, and some other buildings. It was a clear night. We kept the curtains open for a while, even though it seemed as though the people in the apartment across the way could see right in. The nurses who came in thought I was doing really well—handling the contractions, hanging in there. Barbara examined me. I was six centimeters dilated, making progress. I spent most of the first two to three hours in there leaning against the bed and rocking. My legs and feet got tired, but it was the best way for me to handle the pain. Alastair stood next to me and rubbed my back or held my hand, or just stood very close. At some point, Barbara said she thought I was observing myself as well as living through it. She asked me about my novel. (It had been my goal to write a novel before I had a baby.) She sat in a chair and watched us for most of the time. There wasn't much she could do at that point.

When I was dilated to eight centimeters, my labor slowed down. Barbara had two suggestions: She could break my water to try to speed things up, or I could lie down in the position I'd been avoiding, on my side. She was also concerned that my legs were tired from standing up and rocking. Lying on my side was a very painful position, but to me it was an easier solution than having my water broken.

I assumed the hated position, and my labor began to pick up. Now it was getting really uncomfortable. I clutched the top of the bed with my right hand, and Alastair stayed close. The contractions were coming quickly now, and I tried to relax through each one. These were deeper than the others. I hung in there, groaning. An hour and a half later, Barbara took another look and said that I was almost there. She helped me get to 10 centimeters by stretching my cervix. Then my water broke spontaneously.

I don't know what I'd been thinking, but I'd believed that there would be a little break between 10 centimeters and the next phase, pushing. But it wasn't like that. Barbara kept asking me if I wanted to push. Finally I did, or maybe I didn't know what else to do. The pushing contractions were coming fast and furious. Barbara got me into the position she preferred—back cradled, chin down, legs up. She thought that this position helps get the baby down and under the pelvic bone. Barbara held one leg and Alastair took hold of the other, and they pushed my legs toward me. She said I was catching on to pushing, but later I read in her report that it took me a while to figure it out. She would place her finger near my rectum and say, "Push here." It was hard to get the hang of it, to push toward that direction. It was something I had never had to do before.

At one point, Barbara left the room and a nurse helped out. I didn't understand why she stepped out. Probably to rest. It was taking so long. I kept saying, "I'm having a reality problem." I wanted Alastair to calm me down. I think I wanted to stop and take a break, take a rest, reconsider the implications of having a baby. But there was no break, no stopping. My mind waffled around that little room. Alastair got quiet.

When Barbara came back, she took over again. She said, "Judith, don't freak out on me." I listened to her voice, directing me, encouraging. It was my only connection with what was happening. I think I slept during contractions, I was so tired. I'd just fall off in between. I was tired and thirsty and afraid to drink too much. I had some muck in my throat that kept coming up every time I had to push. I swallowed it back, and then took a breath and pushed and pushed. To stop the baby from slipping back, I needed to take a breath, push, and then take a really fast breath and then push again. It took me a while to realize how quick I had to be to get the second push in. Alastair told me later that the muscles in my neck stood out. I was sweating. He kept wiping my face and neck with a cold cloth. I made incredible noises while I pushed, yells from my throat that helped me focus and got the energy in my body in the

15

right place. They were like sounds from a movie. But they did the job. (Later, that morning in my room, I could remember these contractions and how they hurt, but now I can't.)

I kept thinking, "The baby is coming now." Finally they started to be able to see the head. I thought that if they could see the head, the baby must be coming out soon. But it took so long for the head to get down to around the perineum. Finally Barbara started working the perineum, making room, telling me to push exactly where her finger was. This was painful. Every time I pushed I thought, "This is the one, this is the one." And then it wasn't. There were always more to do. I think at some point I just lost it. I stopped thinking about anything except pushing. I didn't think about the room or anything. I was a big old tired pushing machine.

After three hours of pushing, the baby's head began to crown. That was the worst—searing pain through the skin. Barbara had said it would be like someone was tearing you apart. And I guess that's exactly what it was. Then it was like a pop, and the pain was so bad it didn't exist anymore. They had to suction the baby. And then the rest of the baby—a boy— squirmed out. And that was it. I didn't feel anything anymore. I saw his head and his body rush by my bent knees. He had a big head, well-formed features, and clear skin. He looked like a little person. Sam was born at 2:20 A.M. on October 4. (I kept saying, "What time is it," because I wanted to know what day he'd be born. Earlier, around 11 P.M., I was sure it would be October 3.)

They took him away to make sure he hadn't inhaled meconium. This wasn't supposed to happen. He was supposed to be placed right on top of me when it was all over: Bare skin to bare skin. But I didn't really mind. I wanted him to be all right. We waited for him to come back. I pushed out the placenta, and Barbara held it up, a trophy. The cord was a lovely shade of light blue and azure. She showed Alastair and me how it all went together: the cord, the sac where Sam had been (which broke when she held it up). It was amazing. I was sitting in a pool of blood, as happy as could be.

They brought Sam back in, all swaddled up and wearing a little hat. While we were waiting, Barbara kept saying what a big baby he was. When they brought him back, we found out that Sam weighed 9 pounds 10.6 ounces. It was great. Joyous. A big perfect baby! No one could believe how big he was. He just looked at us with clear big eyes. Barbara showed me how to nurse, and he started right in. Alastair got me some orange juice and a sandwich, and I ate half of it. We hung out in that room, me in the blood, until 5 A.M.

The next day, my arms ached, as though I'd been rowing for hours. They ached from holding onto the railing of the bed, straining to push.

I came home from the hospital two days later. I felt like I'd been away for much longer. So much had happened. I looked out the window, at the familiar view, and it looked different. Something had changed. It was me.

❧ 2

Annette's Story

The Home Birth Option

Movement therapist Annette Cantor is used to paying attention to how her body feels and has good instincts about making herself comfortable. There was only one place for her to have a baby—and that was where she was most at ease, at home.

On one side of their small adobe house on Cerro Gordo Street in Sante Fe, New Mexico, Annette and David Cantor have a view of the mountains, and, on the other side, a view of the city of Sante Fe. Annette and David moved there from New York City when Annette was six months pregnant. "When I became pregnant, I got a strong urge to leave the city," said German-born Annette. "I felt as though I wanted to have my baby in an environment that was closer to nature."

Annette never considered giving birth anywhere else but at home, although her husband did. David grew up with a strong belief in modern medicine and later confessed that if it hadn't been for Annette, it would never have occurred to him to have the baby at home.

Home births were part of Annette's family. Annette was born at home in Neuss, Germany, as were three other siblings. During her mother's childbearing years, home births were the fashion, although now the trend in Germany is toward hospi-

18

tal births. Whereas the couple was drawn to Sante Fe because it seemed like a nice place to live, Annette and David were happy to discover that home births were both popular and legal there. (Throughout the United States, home births are mainly performed by lay-midwives, although Annette's midwife was a certified nurse-midwife. The difference between the two is that certified nurse-midwives first become trained as nurses. States have different laws regarding the status of lay-midwives. In some states, they are licensed and legal and often have hospital rights; in other states, they have neither.)

"There are many midwives here, and it's a common practice to give birth at home," said Annette. "Some people say it's for economic reasons: It's less expensive, and lots of people don't have health insurance. So they choose this because it's affordable."

Many women choose to have a home birth because they dislike hospitals. But that wasn't the case with Annette. In fact, she had only good things to say about hospitals. "I had been in a hospital before and had a good experience," said Annette. "I had a bicycle accident in New York City. I was knocked unconscious and woke up in a hospital. My collarbone was broken, and I had a wound in the head. It wasn't major. I had a wonderful experience being taken care of."

Annette's reason for having a home birth was simply that she wanted to have her baby in the place where she felt most comfortable. "It was just generally that I like being at home in my own environment," she said. "Being a movement therapist, I felt that giving birth was my kind of thing. I felt that I would like to have as much freedom as possible to choreograph it [the birth] as I wanted to. I assumed that it would be easier to do this at home than in an institution where there are certain rules you have to adhere to. I never considered anything else."

Annette's confidence stemmed in part from her trouble-free pregnancy and from her background as a movement therapist. Annette specializes in the Alexander Technique, a body-

19

awareness technique in which an instructor helps an individual become aware of how to hold the body and how to correct improper alignment. "The Alexander Technique helped my pregnancy because I was aware of how my body felt and how to take care of myself," said Annette. "Nothing turned into a problem. If I felt tired, I napped. I didn't push myself or pretend that I wasn't pregnant. It is an impulse with me to say, 'Never mind, I can still do a thousand things.' I gave up that attitude and enjoyed pregnancy." Well-nourished and well-rested, Annette felt good.

She made arrangements to have help around the house after the birth, hiring someone to do light cleaning and a *doula* to help with the baby. (*Doula* is a Greek word meaning "mothering the mother, or caregiver of another woman." A *doula* can either help during labor or, as in Annette's case, with postpartum care.)

"Lenya, my midwife, supported what I was doing," she noted. "She helped me remind friends to bring food to our house after the birth. All this made me feel comfortable and I felt surrounded by help and support."

During midwife-run childbirth classes, Annette and David met other couples, some of whom were having their babies in the hospital. "This is the time when I became more conscious of my decision," she said. "In the class, the midwives introduced us to all the things that could happen during childbirth. That's when I started thinking, 'Oh my God. So many problems can occur. Am I making the right decision?' So many women in the class wanted painkillers. I started thinking that I was a lunatic. I went through moments of doubt and fear. And yet the outcome was that I always wanted this birth and it felt right."

Annette got a lot of support from her midwives. "They had a relaxed office atmosphere. With each visit, you'd stay for an hour. They'd check the baby. Their medical procedures were low key, and the rest of the time was spent talking about how you feel, what you're eating, any problems. And so I got the opportunity to talk about my fears. When I got closer to the birth, we talked about what would happen in case I got rude during the birth. They were open to these concerns. I felt as though I had a lot of support. I kept coming back to that. It was my comfort and confidence."

Visits to the midwives' office also gave David a chance to ask questions. "He would sometimes come to the checkups," Annette said. "He would scrutinize the midwife to satisfy his own desire to feel safe. He had many questions about what would happen if something went wrong." As it turned out, the hospital was only 10 minutes from Annette and David's home. "They [the hospital] gave us the feeling that they are open to receiving home births," said Annette. "From talking to other people, we found that they don't make a fuss at the hospital, and the nurses there are used to home births, so they are supportive. That made me feel good, too. If I went to the hospital, I didn't want to feel punished. Truly, in my belief, I was sure I wouldn't have to go to the hospital." And when the birthing class took a trip to the hospital, Annette and David didn't go with them. "I didn't feel it was necessary for me. I deep down believed it would all be really at home."

Annette's due date, May 1, came and went. "Being late presented a bit of excitement," recalled Annette. "By law, in New Mexico, you have to get in touch with a doctor and have a [nonstress] test when you're two weeks late. The whole idea of a home birth is put into question. If the doctor says it's too late and wants to induce you, you have to do that." (The non-stress test determines how the baby and placenta are doing. The baby's heart rate is a good indicator of whether or not the baby is getting enough oxygen and nutrients.)

On the 14th day of waiting, Annette's midwife lent her a breast pump so she could induce labor naturally by stimulating her nipples. It seemed to work. Later that evening, around 11

P.M., Annette began to feel slight contractions. "David finished [putting together] our wedding album. At 11, he wanted to give it to me. I told him I'd look at it tomorrow. I said, 'I need to go to bed because I think it's happening.' "

Annette went to bed and slept. "I had contractions all night," she said. "But I knew I needed to get as much rest as possible. So I was determined. The contractions felt like menstrual cramps, and I just relaxed into them. I think movement awareness helped. I consciously relaxed into them. That helped me spend the night feeling these waves coming and going. I didn't feel concerned or anything. I just felt happy. I was happy and excited that it was happening." And Annette slept through the night until 7 A.M.

When she woke up, she could tell she really was in labor. "I was lying in bed and thinking, 'What's supposed to happen now?' I was very excited at this stage, thinking, 'Oh, this is for real.' " Annette made tea and had cereal for breakfast, while the contractions grew stronger. She thought about telephoning Lenya, but didn't want to call too early. Instead, she waited until 8 A.M., when the contractions were about five minutes apart. "Lenya said, 'It sounds fine. Enjoy your breakfast.' There are different schools of thought about eating while in labor, but Lenya encouraged me to have a nice one and to do whatever I felt like doing—and to make myself as comfortable as possible."

Annette's low-key manner made Lenya respond in kind. "She said she would stop over. My massage therapist, who had also said she would like to be here [for the birth], said she would come over, too."

David had been up until 3 A.M., too excited to sleep. He was sleeping now, and Annette didn't want to wake him. "I called a few friends in New York and told them I was in labor. My parents were on a biking trip for my father's seventieth birthday, so I couldn't tell them. I was a bit sad about it." She took a bath—until about 10 A.M. By then, the contractions were getting more intense, and only a couple of minutes apart. "I felt at that point that I wanted David there. He was still sleeping. I woke him up. He jumped out of bed, all excited."

At about 10:30, Elizabeth, the massage therapist, arrived, candles and oils in tow. And they set up the bedroom, getting it ready for the birth. Annette and David had made preparations ahead of time, sterilizing towels and covering the bed with clean sheets, followed by a rubber cover, followed by more sheets—so the bed could be easily stripped and kept dry during labor.

As the contractions increased in intensity, Annette would stop what she was doing and kneel down or do exercises. Belly dancing helped, as did movement in general. "I did anything that made me feel I was moving, to let the contractions travel through my body." When she wasn't in motion, Annette settled into her bedroom, sitting on the edge of the bed while Elizabeth rubbed her back. "David was there, in a fabulous mood, excited. But from then on, I have no memory of outside events. I don't know if the phone rang. I don't remember what David was wearing or whether he had breakfast. I was focusing totally on the whole process happening to me."

David and Annette spent about an hour and a half together before the midwife and her assistant arrived, at 11:30 A.M. "She came. We made some jokes. She looked at me and washed her hands and said, 'Let's check the cervix.'" Annette was seven centimeters dilated. "It was really happening," said Annette. "Until that point, I was still waiting for more to happen, wondering, 'Is this really it?' Now I knew it was." Lenya went to get her things out of the car. She brought in her doctor's case and oxygen tank, and Annette was interested in looking over her equipment. "It wasn't hectic at all. Everyone was making themselves comfortable. I noticed that I was going more and more inward. I had some water near my bed and had something to drink, but no other food at that stage. I began to really focus in on what was happening to my body. Just being aware of relaxing into the contractions."

Annette tried out several positions, such as squatting or down on hands and knees. But nothing felt as comfortable as sitting on the edge of the bed. Elizabeth and David propped Annette up in bed with pillows so she could lean back, legs spread open wide. David was on one side and Elizabeth on the other. "Lenya was directing us. She kept talking to me, asked me if this was comfortable. Did I want more pillows? Something to drink? The more labor proceeded, the less I wanted. All I wanted was for Elizabeth and David to be next to me and support me, and I held onto them." Elizabeth massaged her back each time the baby pushed down. "David says I had him sitting next to me, holding onto his body for support." Occasionally, someone would put a wet washcloth with lavender oil on Annette's forehead.

"It was a very caring atmosphere," said Annette. "From then on, I imagined the baby moving through the birth canal. Then I got to this place where I have the strongest memory. I felt myself in the darkness in some kind of tunnel, and I saw the light at the end of the tunnel. It went on forever. I had this feeling of being stuck there. I had a great fear somehow. It felt physical. It was painful. I thought, 'I can't do this. This is enough. I can't do more. If I have to, I will burst apart. And I can't allow this to happen. I have to stay together. There is light there, though.' I didn't really have the choice to go through it. I did want to get through it. I just didn't want the pain of going through it. I was very angry. I was swearing to myself, thinking, 'What did I get myself into? I can't do this.' "

Lenya guessed what was going through Annette's mind. "She told me I was doing well," said Annette. "She said it might feel as though I was bursting apart. It's just what you feel like. It just has to open for the baby to come out. I thought,

'Okay, well then.' I heard the others say, 'The head.' The head was starting to come out. I didn't let go."

Because she felt unable to let go, Annette needed lots of pushes to get the baby out. "I was pushing gently," she said. "I had problems holding, coordinating the breathing and knowing when to push. I didn't get it just right at first. Lenya had to show me." Annette pushed for a half hour, although it seemed like forever. "I was really angry. I didn't want to see anything. I didn't want to see the head. I said out loud, 'You stay right here.' I didn't want David to leave. He encouraged me to look at the head and I said, 'Shut up.' "

When Lenya told her to push longer, Annette recalled, "All of a sudden I felt a slipping feeling, something pushing through. I remember them saying, 'The shoulder,' and helping the other shoulder come out. Another push and the baby was out. I heard Lenya say, 'A little girl.' I felt at that moment so relieved. I was crying." They sucked out the baby's mucus and put her on Annette's chest. "I just wanted to hold the baby, put her on my breast. She didn't make much sound. I kept saying in German, '*Masi* [little mouse]. *Masi, Masi.*' Lenya thought I was saying, 'Rosie.' "

Annette was exhausted, but elated, after her seven hours of labor. "I remember this feeling of bliss and happiness, exhilaration right after the birth." Leah was born at three in the afternoon on May 14. Afterward, David told Annette that there had been storms outside during the birth and that they'd had to close the windows and doors. After Leah was born, the storm cleared and it was peaceful outside again.

Naomi, Leah's sister, was born two and one half years later. Naomi was born at home, and Annette's labor lasted about 45 minutes.

❧ 3

BARBARA'S STORY

HOME AWAY FROM HOME AT A BIRTH CENTER

Barbara Cattermole was seven months pregnant with her second child and unhappy with both her obstetrician and the hospital where she planned to deliver. She had to make a change. Just in time, a childbirth instructor introduced her to the Reading Birth & Women's Center.

Barbara Cattermole gave birth to her first child in a hospital outside Philadelphia. Although she'd always been interested in birth centers and midwives, she didn't know of any in her area. "In 1981, the doctor and nurse thought I wasn't behaving properly," said Barbara, a psychiatric nurse. "I wanted to walk around during labor. They wanted me to lie on my left side. They convinced me that I needed pain medication. They told me that they would just give me Demerol. But there was also Thorazine in it, which is a major tranquilizer."

The drugs made Barbara sleepy, and she dozed between contractions. "I hated every minute on drugs," she said. "A contraction would come, and I would wake up. I wasn't prepared to get through it. The medication was worse than the pain.

"Because of the drugs, my son slept for three days after he was born," she said. "I wasn't terribly upset by what happened, and I didn't think I'd had such a bad experience. I'd heard of women who had things happen to them that are much worse than what I had."

Barbara became pregnant again six years later. She was then living near Reading, Pennsylvania, north of Philadelphia, and working as the head nurse at St. Joseph's Hospital. To be loyal to her employer, she decided to go to the hospital's obstetrician and to have the baby at St. Joseph's. "In retrospect, it was a stupid thing to do," recalled Barbara. "The prenatal visits lasted ten minutes. Then I started to go to childbirth classes given by an instructor who also taught at birth centers. During class, she talked about how they deliver babies in hospitals and how they do it in birth centers. My old idea of wanting to go to a birth center and having a midwife came back."

During the pregnancy, Barbara started to reevaluate her decision about delivering at the hospital. A few things happened to make her reconsider. "We went to a sibling party at the hospital for families who would soon be delivering there," said Barbara. "They showed a film about siblings being at the birth. My son, David, wanted to be there. We asked the hospital, and they said, 'Oh, we don't do that here.' " Then "why had they shown a film about siblings being at the birth if the children couldn't do that at this hospital?" Barbara wondered.

Another problem was that the waiting room was a smoking area. "All I could see was my family sitting there for hours, reeking of smoke," said Barbara. "We started to feel a little less positive. I thought, 'This is where I work. I am a nurse. I can control the doctors. I can handle all this.' But I had never looked into all the hospital policies. For example, everyone had to have an IV."

The last straw for Barbara was a disagreement that she had with her obstetrician two weeks before her due date. "I went in for a checkup and he said, 'You look big. You won't be able to use the birthing room.' Then he told me that if I went more than two days past my due date, they'd have to induce labor. I hit a wall. I was upset. People began to worry about me. They thought I would just stay at home and have a paramedic come and deliver the baby. I realized I had no control over the birth. The way they were talking, it felt like I'd end up with a C-section."

Barbara talked to a lot of people. She cried. One day, she was so distracted that she forgot to use her gloves while gardening and got poison ivy all over her body. Luckily, during this time, a childbirth instructor noticed her distress. "She told me about a birth center in Reading," said Barbara. "They were in the phone book, but I didn't even know they were there. I thought there had been a malpractice crisis in Pennsylvania a while ago, and all the birth centers were closed. The center was the same distance as the hospital from me. There *was* a perfectly wonderful option." Barbara found out that the birth center was relatively new and had been open for only a year and a half.

The childbirth instructor called the birth center on Barbara's behalf. She was examined by the birth center's doctor to make sure she met all the criteria for giving birth there. (Birth centers only take women who have low-risk pregnancies.)

Barbara's doctors didn't make it easy for her to leave. "I explained that I was concerned about the direction the birth seemed to be going," said Barbara. "I told him that no one would give me a chance to labor the way I wanted. He said that he would override the orders of the other physicians. But that was ridiculous. I wanted to put my energy into giving birth, not worrying about what my doctors were going to do." When Barbara left, the doctors' practice was in turmoil and split apart shortly afterward.

For Barbara, the Reading Birth & Women's Center was the solution she'd been seeking. The center was a converted house on a residential street with sidewalks and trees. "There were no intercoms or buzzers," said Barbara. "You could hear the birds outside. They had gardens attached to the rooms so you could go outside."

The living room had been turned into the reception area, the dining room was a birthing room, and the kitchen had been left intact. The center had hardwood floors, and a home-like atmosphere. "They had things that people think about at a birthing center, quilts and fluff," said Barbara. "It was like having the birth at someone's home, just not your own."

Barbara went on a tour and orientation at the center, met the midwives, and fell in love with the place—and the philosophy. "I felt more comfortable with the midwives at the birth center two days after I met them than after eight months with the obstetrician," Barbara continued. "It wasn't just the birth center that did it for me. That's just a place where you give birth. It was the midwives' philosophy. They are on your side. You write a birth plan and tell them how you want your birth to go." It was 1988, and the midwives at the Reading Birth & Women's Center didn't have hospital privileges. If a pregnant woman became high-risk, she'd be turned over to the midwives' backup doctor.

The one thing left for Barbara to do was to convince her husband Richard to go along with her. "He had never heard of midwives," said Barbara. "His mother's idea was that only poor people saw midwives. 'What do you mean you're not having the baby at a hospital?' my mother-in-law exclaimed. Richard came with me to the orientation, met the midwives, and saw the place. He was pleased and started to look at birth a whole new way. He even said that, if we didn't make it to the birth center in time, he would deliver the baby himself. The midwife told him he could, but [she] also suggested he catch the baby if it were born at the birth center. And he's a squeamish guy."

The couple's son, David, wanted to be at the birth. This was allowed at the center, but it was recommended that siblings have their own support person to answer questions and look after them. Barbara was pleased with her decision to switch caregivers. Now she could plan to have the birth she wanted, instead of just hoping she would.

A day before her due date, Barbara went into labor. She had contractions all day but didn't tell anyone because she felt comfortable laboring on her own. At about 10 P.M., Barbara called the midwives, and they told her to come in at 11 P.M.

"We got down to the birth center and unpacked," said Barbara. "My son started to play cards. We hung out in the kitchen. I walked around. I was a very happy person. They let me walk, and I love to walk when I'm in labor. The midwives stay with you throughout the birth, so they followed me while I walked. They do whatever exams they need to do, but [they] don't interfere. Having watched so many women labor, they know a lot. My contractions picked up. My water broke and went all over the place. It had a profound effect on my son; he thought it was cool. I had a lot of back labor. It hurt, but I felt safe. There was someone whispering in my ear, 'You can do it.' The midwives don't have you concentrate on breathing, but on visualization—imagine your cervix opening. It made a lot more sense. There were moments when I was scared, but I had people encouraging me. I never doubted myself because I was surrounded by people who knew I could do it.

"The midwife said to my husband, 'If you are the one who is going to catch this baby, you better be over here.' My husband caught the baby and the midwife was right there. David cut the baby's cord."

Barbara pushed for seven minutes. Erin was born at 4:23 A.M., weighing 8 pounds 9 ounces. Barbara's labor had lasted just seven hours. "I like to say that I lay down and had a baby," she said. "I am quick. Born to breed."

Barbara had a small tear and needed a few stitches. "While they stitched me, my husband and son took our daughter to the kitchen. They held her and looked at her. With my first child, I felt detached when he was born. They took him and put him in a warmer. All I could do was look at him from eight feet away. Erin was handed to me. The bonding took place so much quicker. It was important that we all bonded."

Much later, Barbara found out how much catching his daughter had meant to Richard. "We were out, and another man, who had just been at the birth of his kid, had taken pictures and was showing them," said Barbara. "My husband was real quiet. Then he said, 'I was at the birth. I held the baby.' He hadn't just been holding a camera. He held his hands up just as he did when he held our daughter for the first time. You could hear the pride in his voice."

Barbara became pregnant again six years later. From the start, she had her prenatal visits at the birth center. She discovered that the midwives now had hospital privileges. The birth center offered all kinds of classes for Barbara and the family: Self-Care Class, Nutrition Class, Sibling Class, Complications Class (learning what can go wrong during birth and how these issues are dealt with). Richard didn't seem to be involved in the pregnancy, so Barbara wanted to choose female friends as other support people.

Barbara wrote out this birth plan:

We want to keep the birth simple.
Our preference is to have the baby at the Reading Birth & Women's Center.
I want to stay home as long as possible during labor.
Richard will be my coach until it's time to catch the baby.

Our children, David (12) and Erin (6), have chosen to be present at the birth. Becky will be their support person.

I would like to deliver in whatever position seems right at the time.

I really want to avoid an episiotomy.

Richard will catch the baby.

Rosemary will be an all-around support. She will help support Richard and the kids if needed. When Richard is busy catching the baby, Rose can help me. She will also be the photographer.

The baby can nurse as soon as it wants to.

Richard, Erin, and David will have the baby while I am being tended to, i.e., if I need stitches, etc.

We would like time alone as a family to greet our new family member.

We want to go home when the midwife feels it is okay.

My mother-in-law is coming to take care of me and the family for two weeks after the birth.

For Barbara, the pregnancy seemed to go on forever. It was hard for her to juggle her work life and home life while being pregnant. At times, she felt grumpy and unable to keep up with the rest of the family.

On May 23, Barbara started to feel contractions. "Some contractions were stronger than others," she said. "I was able to fall asleep, but woke up at 4 A.M. with contractions that were about eight to ten minutes apart." Barbara put a heating pad on her back. Later the contractions stopped. "I felt like my body was trying to go into labor, but something was stopping it," she said.

At a prenatal checkup the next day, Barbara was three centimeters dilated. She felt contractions all day and evening. By the next morning, they had fizzled out again. On May 26, she was up all night with contractions and passed the mucous plug. Again, when she woke up, the contractions were gone. The labor was so on and off that Barbara told David he could go to Virginia for the weekend to a soccer tournament. And Barbara continued to feel contractions off and on for the next two days. "I was beginning not to understand my own body," said Barbara. "[I thought,] 'Will I know when I'm in labor?' "

Two evenings later, the contractions were unnoticeable, so Barbara went to bed early. "At 2 A.M., the contractions woke me up," she said. "They were about six minutes apart. I could read between them for a while, but they kept getting stronger and closer. I decided that if I still had them at 3 A.M., I'd call the center. I called at 2:55 and told Julie I needed to come in."

Barbara got her family up, and everyone piled into the car. On the way, Richard joked about whether there was time to stop for coffee on the way. "I told him to drive faster," said Barbara. "The contractions kept getting stronger, and my back hurt so much."

They arrived at the birth center at 3:50 A.M. Barbara could barely make it out of the car. "We got inside, and here's where things get a little hazy," said Barbara. "The contractions were so strong across my pelvis and back. They seemed to just come one after the other. I got changed while Richard called Rosemary and Becky, our support people. I kept leaning on the bureau. I felt like I couldn't do it; my back hurt so much. Susan checked me—I was at ten centimeters. I went back over to the bureau to stand. Susan encouraged me to push, and my water broke on the first one. I kept pushing and couldn't stand up anymore. My back just kept hurting."

Barbara lay down on the bed, on her right side. She was aware of everyone at the foot of the bed. "I could feel the head descending with each push," she said. "I could feel the burning. Then I could touch the head. The rhythm slowed. I felt in control. With each push, I could feel the head moving down. After a couple of pushes, the head was out. Next the shoulders. Then Richard placed the baby on my stomach, and there was a lusty cry. I asked Erin to come around and tell me if it was a boy or a girl. It was a boy. All the discomfort and anxiety were gone. It felt wonderful holding him against my skin. He was perfect. We quickly agreed on his name—Alex."

The family went home about six hours after the birth. Richard went to sleep. Erin and Barbara just stared at the baby and talked about the birth. They called their families and David, who had scored two goals in the soccer game that morning. "He said, 'I was right again. I knew Erin would be a girl, and this one would be a boy,' " said Barbara, who was pleased the waiting was over. "Our life is back on track, with one small addition."

4

Ann's Story

An Underwater Birth

*Ann Arscott had always loved water. So it was no wonder
that that was where she wanted to give birth. In England,
where Ann lives, water births are an accepted practice in
many hospitals. Luckily, the hospital's one tub was
available just when Ann needed it most.*

Ann Arscott and her husband Peter live in a small English
village near Oxford. They were married in 1990 and spent
about five years trying to conceive. Although no medical problems were detected, Ann was 36 by that time. It was suggested
that they try in vitro fertilization (IVF). (Eggs are retrieved and
mixed with sperm. When fertilization is confirmed, the embryos are placed inside the woman's uterus.) Their first attempt at IVF worked. "I know other people who go through
IVF, and it becomes the be-all and end-all. 'Will it happen this
time?' they want to know. I would have gone up the wall if I
had not been working at the time."

Ann enjoyed pregnancy. "I had a brilliant pregnancy. I
bloomed. Sometimes I felt tired, but apart from that, hunky-
dory. I even enjoyed being rid of my period for a while."

Ann had always been a swimmer, and her mother was a
swimming teacher. During her pregnancy, Ann swam in the

early mornings two or three times a week, right up to the week before the birth. In a childbirth class, the couple saw a video featuring a water birth. The hospital where Ann planned to deliver, the John Radcliffe Hospital in Oxford, had one birthing pool. Knowing of Ann's love for swimming, Peter asked if she'd consider a water birth. "I hadn't let my hopes get too high," said Ann. "The pool [at the hospital] has to be free when you're in labor. And there have to be no complications. I thought they might see our conception as complicated. If I got all excited and then it wasn't available, I'd be disappointed."

Ann could tell that Peter had been moved by the water birth video. "There was something magical about it," she said. Ann and Peter came up with a birth plan. They wrote it out, and it was put in the folder with their caregiver and at the hospital. "No one makes you do the birth plan. But people recommend that you do it. You talk with your partner about what you want. There's a space in your file for doing it." Ann's birth plan outlined the three main things she wanted:

1. A water birth, if possible.
2. Being examined on the floor and being able to move around during labor, not just lying on a bed.
3. Immediate transfer (after the birth) to Wallingford Community Hospital, a small hospital where Ann would get a lot of personal attention in a relaxed environment.

Ann, who is employed by a foreign-language-textbook publishing company, left work in the middle of June. She was looking forward to a relaxing three weeks before her due date, July 7. "I wanted to do a lot of swimming at a nearby pool and watch [the] Wimbledon [tennis matches] on television," Ann said. "I thought I'd have three weeks of it." But instead, on the morning of June 28, 10 days after she left work, she began to feel funny. "My tummy was upset, and I had some low back pain. I felt different, but I also thought it could be nothing." Peter, who worked in television in London, had arranged to take three weeks off starting in early July. They hoped the baby would be born on time.

Peter went to work, and Ann began to watch Wimbledon. The weather was extremely hot for an English summer, and, because it was too hot to drive, Ann decided to cancel plans to meet a friend for lunch. (Many cars in England don't have air conditioning because it is not usually hot there in the summer.)

"At two in the afternoon, the contractions started," said Ann. "I started recording them and continued to watch Wimbledon. They weren't that uncomfortable. The phone rang, and the answer machine picked up. It was a friend who wanted to know about a hotel. I listened to the message and thought, 'I really must do something about this.' I went to look up the hotel number. I called the friend back. She knew I was pregnant and asked how I was doing. 'I feel funny,' I said. 'Maybe it's starting.' Later, the friend sent me a card and reminded me that I had been in labor then."

At 5:30 in the afternoon, the power went off in Ann's house. "The television went off, and so did the electric clocks. It was odd. Everything is heightened [when you're about to have a baby]. You think that what's going on inside you has an effect [on the rest of the world]." Ann checked with a neighbor and found out that her power was out, too. (Short power outages were common in the village.) After checking, Ann "felt more clearheaded about it."

The next decision was when to tell Peter that labor had started. She had called earlier to tell him the power was off. He worked on shows that broadcast at 6:30 P.M. and 9:30 P.M. So, she called at 6 and asked if he would call back after the 6:30 show. "When he rang, I told him not to panic. I told him to do the 9:30 run and then come right home. It was odd. I wanted to be on my own. I didn't want anyone other than Peter."

Ann continued to record her contractions, and they were getting closer and closer together. "The contractions didn't seem to be indicating anything more," said Ann, who still hadn't called her mother or the doctors. She enjoyed watching Peter's show on television, "which was reassuring." Ann also took lots of bubble baths: "The water thing; I felt much better in the bath." At 7:30, she ate a small meal of chicken broth and yogurt. Ann wasn't that hungry, but she thought she should eat, and, even though it was hot outside, the broth was comforting.

Peter arrived home at about 10:30 P.M. "We slowed things down a bit," said Ann. "He rang the hospital and told them about the contractions. And they said, 'Don't hurry.' Peter had been up early and had had a busy day. He ate some dinner, and we got stuff ready for the hospital. We left at midnight. In the car, the contractions were quite painful. But I never felt as though I'd have the baby in the car."

Twenty minutes later, they checked into the hospital, carrying in a big cushion so that Ann would be able to labor on the floor. A midwife examined Ann. "I was dilated enough to stay in the delivery area. I immediately asked about the pool, and the midwife who examined me said she'd speak to the senior midwife." At about 12:30 A.M., the pool was already occupied. Also, the senior midwife didn't know how busy she'd be—the senior midwife had to be present when the pool was used. If she was dealing with a problem birth, the pool couldn't be used at all.

Ann began to labor in a normal delivery room. "I spent a lot of time on the floor, doing yoga," Ann said. "I sat, knelt on all fours, squatted, used my big cushion. Once I stood up, my water broke." The midwives examined Ann occasionally, but otherwise left Peter and Ann alone. "Peter had brought Mozart's Horn Concerto, and we played it on the cassette player. Peter massaged my back because I had back labor. The midwives provided almond oil. They ask if you want aromatherapy. It helps to take your mind off [what's happening], and it's something nice to smell."

At some point, the pool became available, and Ann and Peter moved to the birthing room with the pool. Ann got right in and stretched out. Her response to the water was, "Bliss, bliss, bliss." Peter had been told he could bring his bathing suit and get in the pool, too. "But when I stretched out in it [the pool], there was no way anyone else could have gotten in," said Ann. "It was bigger than a bathtub and sloped at the back so you have back support. The water was warm, and there was lavender oil in the water."

During the next three hours, Ann was in the water. "It just felt more comfortable. Less weight. We made lots of jokes. I wasn't expecting this, and it was a bit surreal. One joke had something to do with me being a shipwreck."

She received some gas and air through an oxygen mask. "It makes you feel a bit high. It's standard in Britain. It has no lasting effect. I had it most during the last hour. It does take the pain away, and it's something to help you breathe. It helps you to concentrate on breathing. I'd use the mask when a contraction came."

Finally, Ann felt the need to push. The midwife told her to wait. "Waiting to push felt like it was against nature. I had expected the pain of pushing, but not the pain of *not* pushing."

The midwife examined Ann in the water. "They told me I could push. And put a mirror in so that Peter could see the baby's head appearing. I couldn't see much. I usually wear contacts or glasses. When they thought the baby was coming out, they heated up the water in the pool so that she wouldn't be brought into the world in cold water."

Ann pushed for about 30 minutes. "I felt like I was making progress," she said. "It was pain for a purpose. I was stretched out on my back. The midwife caught the baby—a girl—under the water very gently and put her straight onto my breast. You don't have to get the baby out of the water quickly because she is still attached to the cord. She was very clean and very quiet. She nursed a bit straight away. Peter cut the cord. He kept saying, 'Look at this. Look at that.' He commented on her hands, her face, her toes.

"It was easier to push the baby out and odd to push out the placenta," Ann continued. "I felt like I'd done it all. 'What is this about? You want me to do it all over again?' " Rosie was born at 5:53 A.M., weighing 7 pounds 8 ounces.

Ann was pleased that she'd been able to give birth in the water. "I'd experienced the first part of labor on land," she said. "Being able to be on the floor was helpful, but then I'd had enough of that. The water made it different. It was very pleasant. It was a relief and a change of scenery." Ann also realized that she had a relatively short birth for a first labor. It had lasted about 9 hours and 18 minutes. And they had been at the hospital for less than six hours.

As she had proposed on her birth plan, Ann's third request was to be transferred to Wallingford Community Hospital, which has a small maternity ward of four beds. Ann got her wish on that count, too. "They have wonderful support there," said Ann. "I can't say enough good words about it. The hospital where I gave birth is wonderful, but once you are recuperating, there isn't enough staff. I was at the hospital for nearly six hours and had to ask for things."

Ann stayed in the hospital for another six hours after the delivery. Because both she and the baby were doing all right, they qualified to leave the hospital. "Legally, you have to have someone in the car apart from the driver," said Ann, referring to regulations about transferring a new mother and baby. "Most of our friends were at work. We asked a neighbor who worked in the village shop. She came with us."

At Wallingford Community Hospital, Ann could stay for up to a week, but she left after four days. "I had great midwives there," she said. "They helped with breast-feeding. Put essential oils in your bath. They made it special. There is a lovely garden so you can be outside with your baby. Or, at night, the nurses can take the baby away if you need some rest. I was so lucky to have had such a positive experience, first with the water birth and then recovering at Wallingford."

✿ 5

ROSEMARY'S STORY

TWINS NATURALLY

*Natural childbirth and home births were popular in
Rosemary Moore's family. So, even when she found
out that she was having twins, she wanted to give
unmedicated childbirth a try. She wasn't daunted by the
prospect of birthing twins naturally. In order to have the
birth she wanted, she arranged to have plenty of support
and help during labor. It's this support that saw her
through.*

An actor and writer, Rosemary Moore wanted to get her
life together before she had children. She and Josh married
when she was 35, bought a house in Park Slope, Brooklyn, and
began renovating it. Three years later, they decided to have a
baby, and a month after they began trying, Rosemary became
pregnant. Right from the beginning, she enjoyed being pregnant and had a pleasant first trimester.

Rosemary remembers an incident when she was three
months pregnant that should have been a hint of what was to
come. "We were visiting some friends in Washington, and a
family friend exclaimed over [the size of] my tummy. It wasn't
big, but noticeable. You're not supposed to have such a big one
[at three months]."

In January, Rosemary and Josh planned to take their last vacation without children. "We had organized it to have amnio (amniocentesis) the day before we left for Hawaii. 'I guess the amnio will rule out twins,' I said to Josh before we went. I had seen a mother with twins recently and thought she looked like a tragic figure. I had said, 'Don't let that happen to me.' "

They went for their amniocentesis appointment at Beekman Downtown Hospital. Rosemary lay down on the hospital bed and pulled up her shirt, and the technician spread lubricating jell on her belly. "The doctor wasn't there yet, and the technician, who was chewing gum, said, 'Did the doctor tell you there are two in here?' 'Lordy Moses,' I said. These were words I hadn't used since I was eight. I was laughing and crying. I felt guilty. I thought it was my fault. Josh was shocked. He couldn't speak. Finally he said, 'Twice the fun.' "

About finding out she was having twins, Rosemary said, "I was never so surprised in my life, except when I heard my mother had terminal cancer. Nothing is the same afterward."

She was immediately concerned about the babies. "I was so scared when I saw these things in there. I wanted to know if they were okay." The doctor, who had just heard that Rosemary was carrying twins, came in and asked if she and Josh were all right, acknowledging the fact that some parents just want one child. The doctor, who had listened to the heartbeat in the office, hadn't heard two, probably because one of the babies had been under the other. "If you hear one heartbeat, why look for another?" said Rosemary, who thought the doctor was surprised at having missed hearing a second heartbeat.

The doctor began to assess the situation. "She mentioned things like bedrest and a C-section. She was techno-negative. I didn't know this about her. We were upset by her reaction. My sister had her baby at home. My brother's wife is a lay-midwife and had three at home. I had so much support for birth without medication."

They drove home across the Brooklyn Bridge, feeling a mixture of terror and happiness. When they got home, they called their families to tell them the news.

The next day, Rosemary and Josh left for Hawaii as planned. Of course, they talked a lot about having twins and spoke to other people about having twins. "You tell people you're having twins, and they start telling you about the twins they know. There are twins everywhere."

Upon their return from Hawaii, Josh and Rosemary began the task of finding a new practitioner and places to give birth. "We even went for a consultation with a woman who talks to you about options in the city," said Rosemary.

They started at the top of the list and went down. Birth centers and home births were out of the question because of twins. They also took into consideration some of the concerns their original doctor had had, and they acknowledged that having twins could be more risky than birthing one child.

Rosemary and Josh visited two hospitals that were affiliated with midwives. One of the hospitals, St. Vincent's, had its own perinatal facility, which meant that, if the babies were premature (and with twins it was a possibility), they would receive care right there.

As it turned out, Rosemary and Josh also liked the midwifery practice there. "Their policy was that if your pregnancy is normal, you don't need bedrest," said Rosemary. "They had delivered twins before. They didn't predict any problems."

There were only two things Rosemary had to do differently because she was carrying twins. Most expectant mothers in this midwife practice could meet the backup doctor *if they wanted to*. Rosemary *had* to. With twins, the doctor would have to participate in the birth. Rosemary also had to have a sonogram in her sixth month to determine if the babies were growing at the same pace. At that point, she learned that both of the babies' heads were down. "So we had a fighting chance at natural childbirth," she said. "Their heads were down, and it turned out that they stayed that way."

Rosemary wasn't working, and she concentrated on taking care of herself. "In the third trimester, I only did one thing a day, [like] putting up curtains, going shopping. I hauled around, but I also took naps."

In the middle of the third trimester, Rosemary got serious Braxton Hicks contractions and had to slow down. "We put a mattress in the living room. I was on bedrest for two weeks until they stopped. Then I became more selective about my hauling around, but continued. I wanted curtains on all the windows. I wanted lace curtains on the French doors of the babies' room. I was nesting."

Rosemary also got to know the mothers in a local twins group, went to La Leche League meetings to learn about breast-feeding, and hired a baby-sitter. "I did everything I could beforehand," she said. "It was the unknown. Would the babies be premature? colicky?" Rosemary and Josh attended childbirth classes in their neighborhood and met other couples who were also expecting. Later, several of these families would turn out to be good friends.

July 2 was Rosemary's due date. Midway through June, Josh, a composer and musician, started to wear a beeper. "I began getting baby-sitters for myself," said Rosemary, referring to friends who would hang out with her while Josh was working. "I probably wouldn't have done this if I was only having one child. But having twins was like going off in a spaceship. I like being prepared for big things."

On the afternoon of Saturday, June 23, Rosemary did some errands in the neighborhood and felt twinges similar to preperiod cramps when she was walking home. Josh was leaving for work; he was playing at a wedding outside the city. "We called Deborah (Rosemary's brother's wife in California) and asked her if Josh should go to work." The decision was that

45

Josh should go. Meanwhile, Deborah booked a flight to New York so she'd be there for the birth.

Rosemary settled in for the day. She started to watch *Red River* with John Wayne. "I went to the bathroom, and my water broke," she said. "What's the thing you look at when your water breaks? Is it clear? No, mine was brown. That means there's meconium in the water." (*Meconium* is the material that accumulates in the bowel during fetal life and is discharged shortly after birth. If any meconium is discharged when the baby is still in utero, there is a chance that the baby could inhale it into the lungs. This can be associated with breathing problems at birth or the development of pneumonia.) "I called the midwives, and they told me to come to the hospital now," said Rosemary. Rosemary beeped Josh, who had left an hour before, but couldn't reach him. Rosemary's friend Ann was coming over to keep her company. When she arrived, Rosemary opened the door and said, "Ann, it's drama time."

Rosemary was ready. Her suitcase was packed. With Ann's help, she made a checklist and canceled some dates. "I called some family friends [Harry and Gay] who are like godparents. I told them Josh wasn't here. They said they'd come to Brooklyn to get me."

Rosemary beeped Josh again. "He'd just finished playing 'Satin Doll,' and his beeper went off. He thought, 'Why is she calling me?' When I told him, he was in denial. But he did leave the wedding."

Harry and Gay arrived and immediately left with Rosemary and Ann. "It was a beautiful summer evening," Rosemary said. "The buildings were red, and the sky was blue. Harry knows the city and is a perfect driver. I kept thinking, 'Is this labor?' It felt as though I had period cramps. I tried to see a pattern. I was just terrified. I had made a list of affirmations, things I wanted for the birth. I had wanted to labor at home. I had wanted Josh there. I was scared Josh wouldn't come. You're so confused. You've never given birth before."

They drove through Greenwich Village to St. Vincent's Hospital. Gay and Ann went into the hospital with Rosemary while Harry parked the car. Rosemary was shown to a small labor room. "The backup doctor said that if I was in active labor by 11 P.M., I was all right. I was lucky. Most doctors would do a C-section with meconium and my age [which was 39]."

Josh arrived in his tuxedo, his face white. Linda, a close friend and *doula* (labor coach), arrived, still dressed up from a party. Ann and Gay left, and Rosemary's support team, Josh and Linda, took over. When a larger corner birthing room became available, Rosemary was moved. Because of the twins, the staff knew that Rosemary would need more people involved and more equipment (three monitors, two for the babies, one for Rosemary's contractions).

Rosemary's father, who lives in the neighborhood, came to keep her company. She was glad to have him but, after a while, because of the contractions, felt she couldn't talk to him anymore. Her dad, who is a retired bishop, said a prayer and blessed Rosemary. "He looked pretty worried. But it was sweet to have him there.

"You are getting more and more terrified," said Rosemary. "Things are getting eerie. You look at the nurse. The pain is getting kind of bad—although when I look back, it wasn't so bad. You just go on that trip. It's exciting that it's happening. But the biggest thing with a first birth is the unknown. You think, 'This isn't so bad,' and it gets worse. I had asked a friend, 'Is childbirth like having your arm pulled off?' and she said 'Yes.' I was expecting something horrible, the unknown, and bracing myself for the worst. The great thing was I had midwives, Josh, the corner room, and had done my homework. We had our ducks lined up."

By 9 or 10 that evening, the doctor checked in again and told everyone to get a good night's rest. "He had changed his mind about being in active labor by 11 P.M.," said Rosemary. "He would let me labor until 6 A.M."

The pain was becoming more difficult to deal with. Rosemary had back labor, and it took two people to help her. While one massaged her back, the other held her hand. Peggy, the midwife, was in the middle of her shift. She was tired and went to take a nap, and that was fine with Rosemary, Josh, and Linda because they were handling the situation themselves.

Rosemary had spent a lot of the labor in bed. She had been in the birthing room for about three hours, and it was then 11:30 P.M. But her labor wasn't progressing. Linda wanted Rosemary to stand up and walk around, but it was difficult because she was hooked up to three monitors. Josh suggested they get an extension cord, and one was found. Now they could keep an eye on how the babies were doing at the same time that Rosemary moved around. "I didn't do a lot of walking. I ended up sitting on a low stool that had a hole in it, a birthing stool. I spent most of the time on that stool. I was sitting on the stool with my arms and head on the bed. That was my method of coping."

From about midnight until 4 A.M., nothing much happened. Peggy rejoined them at about 3 A.M. And Rosemary's labor went from painful but manageable to painful and excruciating. "It was hard to stay positive," she said. "But, having my support team, I was able to. I think a lot of labor stops because people don't have emotional support. Linda was there, and she was fiery. Josh has dogged determination. We had a commitment to what I could do. All these people were telling me I could do it. You just have to go through it. If you're halfway through a contraction, you're almost through it. It was a Zen thing that I used. And, having been an actress, I was also comfortable making a low growl the entire time:

Ugggggggg—intoning. When the pain got bad, I was in my body like an animal."

The third technique Rosemary used to get through the contractions was to "think of the scariest thing I'd ever done, which was going out on stage to do my monologue shows. I used that experience. The moment before I went on, I was terrified. But I'd pull myself together to face it. I remembered the feeling of going on stage, using that courage."

In between contractions, there were little breaks. "As short as they were, they were everything," says Rosemary. She went to the bathroom often and hugged Josh a lot.

By 6 A.M., Rosemary was in active labor. At 7 A.M., Rosemary's sister-in-law Deborah arrived on the red-eye from California. "She was in her California flower dress and her good attitude. I couldn't open my eyes, but she was a breath of fresh air." She was a registered nurse, and Rosemary thought she'd be able to help.

Time lost significance for Rosemary. "Ten minutes or three hours could take an eternity. I didn't know how I could get through it. *Ice chip, please*—three very strong words. I needed everybody, and I was always holding someone's hand. I had to have people with me at every corner."

One of the main jobs of the support people and nurses was to watch the monitors to make sure the babies' heart rates were all right. And the doctor would pop in and out of the room to see how Rosemary was progressing.

At 10 in the morning, Rosemary felt the urge to push. "Then I'm pushing and pushing. People could spend more time in childbirth class learning to push. Bear down as if having a bowel movement. The nurses were strict about this—chin down—[and] whether or not you should make a noise. I kept wanting to make a noise, and they didn't want me to. The hard part was keeping my legs in the air. I just wanted it to stop. I pushed beyond my outer limits. It was one hundred times past what I thought I could achieve. How could I ever look the same way at a woman who has a kid? 'Don't forget this,' I said to myself. 'Don't forget this.' It's the inner knowledge that is the most challenging experience." Rosemary knew she'd want to remember the difficulty of labor because "it's such an amazing experience, and it's so extreme."

When Rosemary first started to push, there were several people in the room, including three nurses and a few pediatricians. "The nurses were the most wonderful people in the universe," said Rosemary. "They encouraged me. What a job! You're at the edge of the abyss, and they just stick with you. I really needed their guidance."

Rosemary began to push out the first baby. "The baby's cord was too short. It wasn't my bad pushing. The baby kept snapping back in. They asked if I wanted a mirror. I said no. I just had to concentrate. And then the baby came out—and it was a girl, Faye. That was wonderful." It was 1:15 P.M.

While Rosemary was pushing Faye out, the backup doctor held the other baby in place. With more room in the uterus, there was a chance the second baby could turn and end up breech.

Rosemary couldn't stop to celebrate Faye's birth; she had to have another baby. "I enjoyed Faye's birth, but the exhaustion and pain took away from it—it wasn't rational, but I couldn't relax. I was excited but had to remain in my meditative state. I said, 'Oh, good,' and closed my eyes again. I'm someone who can hardly say hello when I'm under a deadline. I wasn't going to be happy until all was done. I was like a long-distance runner."

Rosemary held Faye for a little while, and then she was taken away. "Because she was a twin, she had to be resuscitated," said Rosemary. "I wanted to get the second one out." Rose expected the second baby to follow Faye right out, but it didn't. " 'Can't you get this baby out?' I said to the doctor. And he said, 'You can't close up shop now.' " As it turned out, the doctor had to do a C-section across the hall, so he let Rosemary continue to labor.

"I went back to eight centimeters," said Rosemary. "They gave me Pitocin. You thought you were on the edge before. Your body isn't your own anymore. Your body is a blob. They are pressuring you. They're trying to be nice, but you just have to do this. There's sweat all over you. Your body is all open. There are a million people in the room. The inside of your body is there for the taking. They're checking you."

Rosemary didn't like the Pitocin. "Pitocin hurt like hell. It's like an unnatural labor contraction. It made the contractions come strong, too strong, and then the baby's heartbeat went down. Something wasn't right. They took me off Pitocin."

Rosemary went to the bathroom again. "I don't know why I wanted to go. I went with Josh. And there was something about that. I wanted to stay on the toilet. It was a small bathroom. Josh was holding my hand. It was like escaping, an attempt to get out of this."

It was one and a half hours after Faye's birth. Linda, who was half asleep herself, was holding Faye. "Before the Pitocin, they asked if I wanted to nurse Faye. They thought it would get the oxytocin going. [*Oxytocin* is the hormone that causes labor to begin; it's also the hormone that triggers the milk to come out when you breast-feed.] I wish I had spent more time with Faye and nursed her, but I was too miserable."

Finally, Rosemary was back to 10 centimeters and pushing again. "I would have gone for anything [any kind of intervention] then," she said. "But they thought I could do it." Rosemary kept pushing, and finally the baby started to come. "There was trouble because the baby was face up and the cord was around it. The nose was mushed."

Rosemary and Josh thought the second baby was going to be a boy. But they were more than delighted to find themselves with two girls. Violet was born at 4:05 P.M. and weighed 5 pounds 2 ounces. Faye weighed 6 pounds 3 ounces. "Who would have thought that there would be three hours between babies?" was the question Rosemary asked afterward. (In most cases, twins are born within 10 to 30 minutes of each other. But it's not unusual to have contractions slow down after the first baby is born.)

"I was done," said Rosemary. "I had a drink. It was the best. By that time, there were zillions of people in the room: pediatricians, residents, nurses, the backup doctor, midwives. It was a big room. They wrapped up the babies, and I held them. My dad and his wife came in. A million people in my family were outside waiting.

"It had been so exhausting and demanding that the babies were an afterthought. I just wanted to rest. I liked holding them but didn't mind them being taken away to get washed up. I wished someone had talked to me more about the time when they came out. If someone had prepared me, I would have been able to hold them longer. You want to be able to hold them."

Rosemary was wheeled to her room, and the babies were brought to her. "We were so happy and so proud," she said. "We had everything we wanted. We'd been lucky because both babies had been head down and stayed that way. We had educated ourselves so we knew what to expect. I had talked to other mothers of twins. I wasn't twenty-two. I was ready."

After three nights in the hospital, Rosemary, Faye, and Violet went home. Rosemary explained that if she hadn't had twins, she would have liked a second pregnancy. "But we never had to talk about it. I think I did it the easy way."

PART TWO

There's Nothing Wrong with Help— Births with Painkillers and Epidural Anesthesia

✤ 6

JOANNA'S STORY

A MEDICAL BREAKTHROUGH

*It was a medical miracle that Joanna Allen could conceive
and carry a baby to term. There was no part of labor she
couldn't handle. But it was during her second birth that she
had the experience she'd always dreamed about.*

When Joanna Allen and Jeffrey Lodin began trying to conceive, little did they know that they were setting off into an unknown world of medicine. For Joanna and Jeffrey, having a
baby was more complicated than it is for most people. "I had
to go through a lot," said Joanna. "Getting pregnant was half
the battle."

Two years after they began trying, Joanna still wasn't
pregnant and they consulted a doctor. "The first thing they do
is take a complete gynecological history," said Joanna, who
knew she had an irregular menstrual cycle, an indication
of a hormonal imbalance. "They did the least invasive thing
first. I had an X ray of the uterus and tubes. They could see a
problem there." Joanna had an unusual uterus, a unicornuate uterus—only one side of her uterus was developed,
and it was half the normal size. It also meant that she had only
one functioning fallopian tube. "The unicornuate is pretty
rare," said Joanna. "My doctors didn't know the capacity of
mine; some women have thirty percent capacity, others

have seventy percent. In some cases, it's possible to carry a pregnancy."

Laparoscopy (a surgical procedure in which a small optical device is inserted into the abdomen allowing the physician to look inside) confirmed that Joanna's uterus had diminished capacity of about 50 percent. "When I had surgery to confirm the unicornuate, they also confirmed that I had one good tube that was healthy," said Joanna. "As I went under, there were about seven other doctors in the room watching the procedure. They don't often get to see this kind of uterus. They were looking at it to get experience. The pictures are in a textbook somewhere, full color."

Because of the hormonal imbalance and the size of her uterus, Joanna was put on Clomid, an estrogen-type drug that stimulates ovulation, at the same time that she was inseminated via her working tube. She tried this for ten cycles. "The whole process of determining when ovulation was about to occur was time-consuming and cumbersome," said Joanna. "Every cycle, Jeffrey would have to go there [to the lab] to ejaculate, and I'd go later to get inseminated. It was a whole-day affair. One day, I went down to Jeffrey's studio and brought a jar and then ran it to the lab. It was like a scene from a movie." After being inseminated, Joanna would rush home in a cab. "I'd try to lay down in the cab. Everyone [who is inseminated] does it. Gravity is working against you. When I got home, I'd keep my hips in the air for as long as I could until dinner time or until I had to get up. Maybe two or three hours. I would lay on my right side [the side where her good fallopian tube was] for hours."

It became "depressing and frustrating," said Joanna, who got tired of tracking her ovulation and buying ovulation kits each month. "It wasn't just a stick in urine. It was more involved. You had to time it and make chemicals. It was a cumbersome process."

The next level of insemination method is *gamete intrafallopian transfer* (GIFT)—eggs are put with sperm into the fallopian tube. When the doctor suggested that Joanna and Jeffrey try GIFT, they agreed enthusiastically. "There was no question that it [GIFT] wouldn't work," Joanna said. "I always felt in my heart that the sperm and eggs were not getting together. Because GIFT takes the eggs and sperm and injects them together into the fallopian tube, it boosts conception one extra step. I had a lot of faith that we would conceive."

After only one try with GIFT, Joanna conceived. She could almost feel the conception happening. "It was such a happy day," said Joanna. "We both felt really great."

Joanna had been reading about pregnancy and childbirth throughout her infertility treatments. "During the course of these treatments, I read everything I could get my hands on. I was feeding my baby hormone. I read midwifery and obstetrics textbooks. My dream had been to have a nonmedicated birth in a birthing center with a midwife. But once we knew I was high-risk, we knew we couldn't. But we wanted to retain as much of that experience as we could."

Joanna was recommended to a high-risk medical group. "I made it clear to them—I wanted it natural. I wanted a labor support person or a midwife there. They said, 'Whatever you want.'"

Because of her high-risk pregnancy, Joanna had to see her obstetrician every two weeks. "Because I went so often, I got to know all the doctors and nurses," she said. "They became like family. I knew I was being treated like a medical anomaly, but the bottom line was that I trusted them completely. They listened to me, too. They knew that when they sent me home, if I felt any symptoms, I'd call them. The trust was mutual. I think that was the key to the whole experience."

Joanna was given a *cerclage* when she was in her 12th week. (A *cerclage* is a string and button that is stitched into the cervix, at the opening, to ensure that it stays closed.) "It was preventative," Joanna said. "It was anticipating a problem. They didn't want me to go through a pregnancy and lose it."

From the 20th week on, twice a day Joanna had to put on an at-home electronic fetal monitor in the form of a belt and check herself. If she had more than six contractions in an hour, there was the possibility that it could turn into labor. If there was the slightest hint of labor, Joanna knew exactly what to do: "I had to force fluids and lie on my side. I drank eight twelve-ounce glasses of water." Joanna explained that hydration would stop the contractions and that the slightest dehydration could cause the uterus to contract. Joanna also lay on her left side to take the pressure off the uterus and allow the baby to get more oxygen.

Once, during the 30th week, Joanna had a scare. The contractions kept coming. She had been given a drug to take to stop the contractions if that happened. The drug would relax the muscle. "The drug was for emergencies," said Joanna. "This time, I had to take the drug and monitor it until I was able to stop the contractions and get it under control."

At exactly 37 weeks, Joanna's water broke. "I knew I had to get the cerclage out. I couldn't labor at home at all. I would have torn. My contractions came quickly, every five minutes." Joanna and Jeffrey went to the hospital. By 10:30 at night, labor was definitely underway. "It had already been a long day. I was tired already. When the obstetrician took out the cerclage, it was the most pain I'd ever had in my life. The baby's head was pushing on the cervix, and the doctor had to push the head over to take out the stitch. There was no time to give me anything. That was really bad. That took a lot out of me. I was still having contractions. The doctor would wait to push the baby's head aside between contractions."

The doctor used what Joanna described as "medieval instruments to push him back up. They had to push against the contractions and against the baby." She said that even at age three and one-half, Joey had a tiny indentation on his forehead from that part of the labor.

After the cerclage was out, Joanna labored for four hours on her own. "I had back labor. The contractions were coming quickly. I didn't have much time to rest in between. I tried to get on all fours and get pressure off my back, but I wasn't successful. I tried walking and squatting and finally asked for an epidural."

It took a little while to prepare the epidural, to hydrate Joanna, and to put in the IV. "Once they got the epidural in, there was some relief. It took the edge off. But it also slowed down the labor. At about 4 A.M., Joanna was four centimeters dilated. "I watched the sun come up over Central Park. At 7 A.M., I was at four and one-half centimeters."

The doctor put an internal monitor on the baby and checked his blood-acid level. "At 7, the doctor said, 'We have 20 minutes.' He [the baby] was in stress. He wasn't distressed yet, but he wasn't being oxygenated. And his heart rate was dropping and not getting back up. The doctor said, 'Get the operating room ready.' They gave me oxygen and told me to lie on my right side, and he checked me."

In the next six minutes, Joanna dilated from $4\frac{1}{2}$ to 10 centimeters. "There were a lot of people in the room at that time, residents, nurses, Jeffrey. 'Let's let her push,' the doctor said. I gave two pushes, and he got out the forceps. They wanted him out. The cord was pressed up against the side of his head, cutting down on his oxygen. Once they saw the cord there, they wanted him out."

Because of the anesthesia, Joanna was not aware of the forceps. "I did my pushes. I saw him take his 'spoons' [forceps] and felt the warmth of the baby slipping out. He was put right on me. I kept saying, 'Is he okay? Is he okay?' There were about eight people in the room, but it felt like twenty. They were prepared to resuscitate the baby if necessary, but he was crying. He was breathing. The nurses said, 'He's fine, he's perfect.' " Joey was born at 7:13 A.M., 13 minutes after the doctor had said the baby had to come out. "It happened very fast. My first sensation was gratitude. It wasn't my fantasy, but the result was the same. Jeffrey looked at me and said, 'Would you do it again?' And I said, 'Yes, in a second.' "

Asked if she was treated differently because of her medical condition, Joanna said she didn't know because she hadn't been through a delivery before. "My body was in shock. I lay there staring, in shock from it. I didn't experience this the second time, the emotional impact of it. 'Oh my God, he's here and I'm a mother. What do we do now?' "

Joanna and Jeffrey had always wanted a large family, and often talked about having four children. Because of this, they had been sure to freeze embryos for future conception. "When I conceived through GIFT, they retrieved twenty-five eggs. We used six to conceive Joey. Then we had the rest put back in the freezer. When we decided to conceive again, we had seven and used five to conceive Christopher."

Baby number two was conceived on January 1 in the hospital. "It's like insemination," said Joanna. "It's timed with the natural cycle, using ultrasound, on the right day. It's done like a pelvic exam." As it had been with Joey's conception, this was another happy day for Joanna and Jeffrey.

During the second pregnancy, Joanna didn't have to monitor her contractions twice a day. But she did have contractions again—contractions even earlier than 20 weeks. "There were contractions, but I was educated, more aware. With Joey, it was preventative. With number two, they loosened up. My doctor felt that I had the experience. Every time I went in, we discussed the monitor. He looked at the pattern of my contractions. Except for that one scare, I hadn't had a lot in one day." When she did have contractions, Joanna did as she had done before—she drank fluids and lay on her side. She could always control them herself.

At 31 weeks, Joanna took Joey to his play group, and her water broke. "Even though it was just a leak, I knew what it was." Joanna went to her doctor's office, and Jeffrey took over at the play group. The doctor confirmed that amniotic fluid was leaking. "They measured the baby to see how big he was and what his heart rate was, to see if he was recovering from the contractions. I knew he was okay. He was still pummeling me. He had always been active in utero."

The doctors let Joanna and Jeffrey make the decision about what to do. Some of the doctors thought they should take the cerclage out and see what happened. "The older doctors felt I could hold on for a while. He'd be closer to five pounds. We knew he was at least four pounds from calculating the length of his bones. He was big for that gestational state," said Joanna. "Many babies are two or three pounds at that stage."

But there was some risk involved. "The problem was infection," said Joanna, "when the water breaks and you wait. But the doctors thought the break in the uterus was high. Every day was a few more ounces for him. The bigger he was, the better."

The doctors laid out what might happen. If Joanna became infected, she could have a sick baby and possibly have to have a C-section. Having the cerclage didn't help because it was a foreign body. "Knowing all this, we decided to wait," said Joanna. She went home and had to lie down on her back, drink a lot of fluids, and take her temperature frequently to check for fever (a sign of infection). She went to the doctor's office every day to have her white blood cells counted. The whole time, she leaked amniotic fluid. "They measured how much fluid was in there for him, and there seemed to be enough, and he continued to produce it."

A few days later, Joanna felt stronger contractions. "I felt like I was going into labor," she said. "I couldn't stop these contractions with rest or fluid. I called my doctor. I had held out for three days." Joanna met her doctor at the hospital at six in the evening. He took out the cerclage. This time, it wasn't as painful. Joanna wanted to know if she could go back home.

"They told me I was having the baby tonight," she said. "They knew once the cerclage was out, it would go quickly. The doctor told me that when I felt like I couldn't take it to call him. He knew as soon as the contractions became intense it would happen. It was a small baby, a second pregnancy."

At first, Joanna sat in her bed at the hospital, looking at a magazine. The residents and nurses kept looking at the monitor. Soon, Joanna stopped looking at the magazine. The contractions were getting more intense. "I could tell we were moving quickly. Between contractions, I was almost stoned. I felt like I was drugged. I was just trying to breathe and get through them, to concentrate on anything—the clock, the monitor. I knew I was close, and I'd gone over that threshold. I said, 'I'm going into transition.' When a nurse told me that my contractions were not so strong and that I was only at four centimeters, I almost barked at her to get the doctor."

He got there in 10 minutes. " 'I think I need some help,' I said to him. I was lying on my left side, staring at a piece of equipment. I found a dial that was my focal point. I thought I was inside and outside my body." They checked Joanna, and she was at eight centimeters. There was no time for any medication. The baby could come before the anesthesiologist could even walk into the room.

Because there were no birthing rooms free, Joanna was wheeled into the operating room. On the way there, she felt the baby slide into position. " 'I have to push,' I screamed, and they looked at me. 'Don't push,' they said. That was the hardest part. It was the most overwhelming sensation not to do it when I really wanted to."

When they got Joanna to the operating room, she gave two or three pushes. "It was the best. Once I was able to push, it was the biggest relief." Christopher was born six minutes from the time Joanna was at eight centimeters and was placed immediately on her. "Once he was screaming, I knew he was okay. He needed a little support, but everyone was very relaxed. It wasn't an emergency." Christopher weighed 4 pounds 6.5 ounces at 31½ weeks.

When she was pushing, Joanna had been given an episiotomy because a premature baby's head is soft and can be damaged by the passage out. The episiotomy also gives the fragile baby more room to come out. "Being given Novocaine and being stitched up was unpleasant, but it was minor. I could care less."

Christopher was taken to the neonatal intensive care unit. Joanna was more concerned about the baby's health than her own. "If he had continued to grow, he would have been twelve pounds at birth," she said. "For a premie, he was a big one. But I'd take a big baby and a C-section over a premie. It's hard to see your baby with tubes in an isolate or incubator, being fed intravenously. You can't hold him and can't nurse. It's not a way to start life. I'd rather take it on myself. He didn't understand. But we were lucky, he was only in for ten days. Compared to other babies in the ICU, he was huge, a giant."

Joanna pumped breastmilk at night to bring him a feeding during the day. He was sleeping all the time so he wasn't awake enough to suck through a bottle. Instead, he was fed through a tube in his nose that went to his stomach. "He was incubated for two days to help him breathe," she said. "He had to burn a lot of calories in order to breathe. He didn't gain weight right away because he slept so much. Once he was over five pounds, he started eating a lot."

It was hard for Joanna to go home without her baby. But she and Jeffrey were thrilled when they could bring Christopher home. On the day that was supposed to be his birthday, he weighed 6 pounds.

"Christopher's birth was the most thrilling and exhilarating experience in my life," said Joanna. "The high lasted for weeks. I felt as though I was filled with natural endorphins going through my body. It gave me a lot of strength, especially in those early days [when he was in the hospital], and I was doing the hospital shuttle."

❦ 7

MIRIAM AND TIM'S STORY

LEARNING ABOUT THEMSELVES AND EACH OTHER DURING A LONG LABOR

Although they had planned for an unmedicated birth, Tim and Miriam discovered that over the course of Miriam's 52-hour labor, they needed different drugs to help them through. While Miriam did not have a good experience with Nubain, a synthetic narcotic, she did have "a beautiful birth" with the help of an epidural.

Tim Standing and Miriam Block of Oakland, California, often talked about how their marriage was a partnership. They imagined that Miriam's pregnancy would be the same way. But, during the first trimester, it wasn't. They felt separate from each other and weren't working together. A few weeks into the pregnancy, Tim surprised Miriam with a trip to Europe. Her parents lived in Belgium, and it was arranged that the two couples would go to France together. Miriam began to experience morning sickness a few days before they were to leave. Under ordinary circumstances, she would have been excited about going, but she was feeling unsettled and was afraid of losing the baby. "It was

65

hard for me," said Miriam. "He told me the day before we left. I was just holding on, knowing what I could eat at home."

Once in Europe, jetlag and morning sickness set in for Miriam. "I grew weaker and weaker," she said. "I couldn't keep anything down." Tim felt unappreciated for arranging the vacation. His goal of giving Miriam a wonderful gift hadn't worked. Miriam spent the whole trip to Paris in bathrooms.

They hoped Miriam would feel better when they got back, but the nausea continued. She couldn't do anything and was throwing up twice a day. She lost eight pounds during the first trimester. Tim wanted to help and did all the cleaning, laundry, shopping, and cooking, always trying to find foods that would agree with Miriam. But there was nothing he could do to ease her discomfort. She hung out in bed most of the day, sleeping and throwing up, while Tim took care of the household. "She seemed to be hostile," he recalled. "There was nothing I could do to help. I was trying to be superdad." Finally, he decided he wasn't going to do it anymore.

At about this time, Tim had to go away on a business trip. "When I came back, Miriam had spent ten days without me," he said. "Her attitude had changed." Tim and Miriam began to work together. She made him feel appreciated and gave him feedback so he could be supportive.

Although she'd felt healthy before she became pregnant—swimming and taking vitamins—pregnancy didn't agree with Miriam. "I love the way I looked pregnant," she said. "I carried in the front, like a big basketball. It was very pretty. But I felt terrible."

Although Miriam had always thought she'd want a home birth, when it came down to planning, she opted for a doctor and a hospital. Miriam didn't relish the idea of a tense, winding, downhill 15-minute ride through the hills of Oakland in winter if a home birth didn't work out. So instead, they planned to deliver at Alta Bates Hospital in Oakland.

Miriam had a female doctor she liked, with whom she'd had minor surgery. When Miriam first started seeing her, she was in practice with midwives. But as the pregnancy progressed, the doctor's practice changed. The new practice didn't include midwives but did include many doctors. "Every month, we'd have six appointments with six different doctors," said Tim. It became less and less likely that Miriam's favorite doctor would deliver her. Still, they decided to stay with the practice. "The changes in her practice were disappointing to me because we realized that we might not get her," said Miriam. "But I trusted her as a surgeon, therefore, I trusted the people she was associated with."

Because the doctor no longer worked with midwives (who would stay with Miriam throughout the labor), Tim and Miriam decided to get a *doula* (in this case, a woman who would be a labor-support person or coach). Linda, the *doula*, was helpful before the birth. She advised them to be flexible, helped them write out a birth plan, and suggested ways to avoid an episiotomy. Linda also gave them guidelines about laboring at home. She'd monitor Miriam by phone until the contractions got so painful that Miriam couldn't talk through them. Then she'd come over.

Their birth plan went like this:

We don't want Miriam to be offered pain relief unless we request it.

We want the baby to receive *oral* vitamin K. (Giving newborns vitamin K is routine at many hospitals, and it is often given as a shot.)

We want the baby's first Apgar test to be performed on top of Miriam.

We don't want the baby to be suctioned unless it is necessary.

"We wanted to go as natural as possible," said Miriam about the birth plan. They were counting on Linda to help them in the hospital. If a doctor they didn't know came in, they would rely on Linda to tell them if they were being "given a line." Tim would be better able to take care of Miriam while Linda made sure the baby was all right or made suggestions about Miriam's position. "Linda was someone who knew birthing," she said. "She knew the routine. She could help us manage the whole situation."

"I was glad she [Linda] was going to be there," added Tim. "We are expected to be experts, and we're not. I had to tune into Miriam and wanted to experience the birth myself."

Tim and Miriam toured the hospital and liked what they saw. The birthing rooms at Alta Bates were like motel rooms. There wasn't much equipment, except for a fetal monitor. Tim and Miriam could have as many people or things in the room as they wanted. Tim would be able to take showers with Miriam, and he wasn't required to wear a bathing suit.

Tim and Miriam took birthing classes. Miriam, who had spent a lot of time doing meditation, felt confident that she'd know how to breathe through the pain. During their childbirth classes, they saw two videotapes of unmedicated births. "I saw these two uncomplicated births and projected from these," said Miriam. "My expectation about birth was that it would be pretty nonstressful. The ride down the hill [to the hospital] would be uncomfortable. But I figured that Nina would have her ride and I'd have mine." (Tim and Miriam found out, after having amniocentesis, that the baby was a girl. They decided to call her Nina.)

Miriam envisioned a six-hour labor, "humming through the contractions. The beautiful birth—I knew it would hurt, but I'd feel the passage of the baby and it would be a spiritual experience."

Tim, on the other hand, expected the birth experience to be difficult. "What happened was not far away from what I expected," he said. "Too many people said that giving birth was like being hit by a truck, and having the most pain they ever felt. I thought that would be hard."

Miriam's due date was January 15. At midnight on January 10, she began having contractions, one every 10 minutes. Miriam and Tim lay in bed together. "The contractions weren't bad," said Miriam. "It was nice to be lying down with Tim, the process starting." Miriam went through the night timing contractions. She couldn't sleep and didn't want to eat because she was worried about having something in her stomach during active labor.

The next morning, the contractions dropped off. "We sat around, wondering what was going on," said Miriam. Tim cleaned up the house, and Miriam went for a walk. She called Linda several times and was told to call her back when the contractions became regular, between five and six minutes apart. But instead of speeding up, the contractions slowed down, dropping down to 7 and then 12 minutes apart.

The next evening, the contractions started up again. Tim went to bed, and Carol, Miriam's mother who had arrived from Belguim for the birth, stayed up with Miriam. It was the second night that Miriam was up and in labor, not eating.

Miriam called Linda every two hours. Some contractions were 5 minutes apart and 45 seconds long. Linda couldn't really tell how Miriam was progressing. She wanted to check her. They decided to meet at the hospital because it was halfway for both of them. Tim called the doctor, and he agreed to meet them at the hospital. "He was very responsive as soon as we said we had a *doula*," said Tim. They left for the hospital at midnight.

As Miriam had imagined, it was painful having contractions in the car, driving on the twisting roads. But in retrospect, she realized that when she got to the hospital, she was feeling pretty good. Miriam was examined in one of the

69

birthing rooms, and a fetal heart monitor was put on the baby. Miriam was only one centimeter dilated. Miriam began to get the shakes (which is common for some women during labor). Linda, who had met them at the hospital, suggested Miriam get in the shower to see if she could warm up and get labor going. Linda realized that Miriam's shakes were the result of nerves. Once Miriam realized that she was tensing up, she understood why; she had been anxious being examined by nurses she didn't know. "By telling me that I was tense, she [Linda] put me in control of it. I could stop shaking then." It was decided that Miriam would be better off laboring at home.

They went back to the house, and Linda went with them. At home, Miriam's mother and Tim went to sleep. Linda and Miriam stayed up, although Linda dozed. "I just continued to have contractions," said Miriam. "They got worse. I couldn't sit down. I spent that night walking around. Between contractions, I wouldn't feel pain. During them, I had back pain." Linda massaged Miriam's back, or Miriam got in the shower. "I'd rock through each contraction," she explained.

By 8 A.M., Miriam was tired. She had now been up for two nights. The contractions had become more painful. Linda could tell labor was progressing now, and she told Miriam it was the right time to go back to the hospital.

While they were waiting for their room at the hospital, Miriam could hear a baby crying—either being born or having a bath. "I thought, 'What have we got ourselves into?' " Then she felt a gush between her legs, and some water came out. The doctors examined the water to make sure it was amniotic fluid. Because it was only a small amount of water, the doctors determined that the amniotic sac had broken high up. Miriam was given another pelvic exam. It turned out that she was only three centimeters dilated. "It was devastating," she said.

This time, Miriam was admitted to the hospital. The doctor wanted to break Miriam's water all the way, in order to help labor progress. Afterward, she stood up because another contraction was coming, and she noticed that she was bleeding. "Everyone looked at everyone else," she said. "No one did anything. They just said, 'We'll just monitor this.' In retrospect, I think they could have freaked out at that point."

It seemed to Miriam that she bled a lot, but she was glad that they let her continue to labor. No one, including the doctor or the *doula*, knew what caused the bleeding.

Throughout the morning, Miriam drank a lot of juice and took showers, while the contractions became more painful. "I was just exhausted," said Miriam. "I didn't think I could make it. I'd been walking the whole time." Miriam had been in labor for about 36 hours and began to think she might need something for the pain. She was tense and couldn't relax. The nurse suggested Nubain, a synthetic narcotic, that could ease the pain. It was also suggested that Tim and Miriam consider an epidural. "I don't think we glared at the nurse, but we didn't want it yet," said Tim. Linda also thought Nubain was a good idea for Miriam. They were told the drug would last from three to four hours, that Miriam would still be able to feel labor, and that it would not harm either Miriam or the baby.

About getting Nubain, Miriam observed, "I was high for hours afterward. It made me feel like I was getting contractions from Kmart." Tim explained, "She felt like someone was buying her contractions from Kmart, sending them, and they were arriving in her body. She was so disconnected. She kept asking me why we were in the hospital."

Miriam sat in the shower, and Linda stayed with her. "I didn't know what I was doing," Miriam said. "I kept asking what these things were I was having. They kept telling me I was having a baby. I thought I needed a strategy. Linda told me I needed to sleep. But I wasn't going back in that room. The

71

contractions woke me up and hurt more when I was out of the shower. It was awful. I was so far removed from being in labor."

Miriam was in the shower for about four hours. During this period, Tim went through an array of emotions. First, he felt left out. "I felt displaced by Linda, shut out," he said. "I was powerless. It was something beyond my control. I realized then that this labor was going to take a long time."

Tim didn't know what to do with himself and tried to think of how he could help. Finally, he decided to go out and buy some food for Carol, Linda, and himself to give them energy for the next few hours. He decided on bagels and cream cheese because the smell wouldn't offend Miriam. During the walk to the store, Tim had a revelation that he later wrote about:

> It was 4:00 in the afternoon and Miriam had been in labor for 37 hours. Carol, Linda, and I had been in the hospital for 7 hours without even thinking of the fact that we might need a meal. I decided it was time to get everyone something to eat, both to make up for the missed lunch and because I knew it would be a long night ahead. We would need all the strength and stamina we had to be there for Miriam and help her through the increasingly intense contractions and the delivery which lay ahead.
>
> Walking down the street, the world seemed very different. I was being very careful crossing the street, waiting for the light, not trusting any drivers on the road. This all seemed like a natural new part of becoming a dad, making sure to take really good care of myself so I could take care of this little one who was coming into the world—a new spirit who I would help guide through the trials and excitement of life, a daughter I

knew I would have to protect until she was old enough to protect herself.

On the way back, I thought about the first conversation I had with Miriam about kids. It was our second date, and I wanted to make sure she understood how much I didn't want children. I knew how strongly I felt about her and wanted to make sure our new romance wouldn't come to a crashing close when she found out how I felt about being a father. Miriam said that having a child with someone was the ultimate expression of love for that person. When two people cared so much for each other, they wanted to create a new person which was part of each of them.

Walking back to the hospital, with my sack of bagels and cream cheese, I finally really felt in my heart the feeling Miriam had described four years earlier. I now know she is right.

Tim went back to the hospital, his spirits revived. Miriam was still out of it. It was as though she had "smoked too much hash or drunk too much," said Tim, who was "determined to stop feeling powerless." While Miriam was in the shower, Tim stood outside, half in, getting wet. He directed the water on her, rubbed her neck and told her to release her shoulders. He was pleased to find that his words and his touch had an effect on her. "I could say something to her and feel with my hands that she recognized me," he said. "In spite of her being out of it, I could reach her."

Said Miriam, "I remember the warmth of his hand, and I focused on that in order to relax. I was in the worst pain I had ever been in."

"Miriam would say one thing, and I would know what to do. It was a great milestone," said Tim, tracing it back to the teamwork they had established when he came home from Boston. In the delivery room, it became clear to him what his relationship with Miriam was all about. "We were doing things together," he said. "We weren't keeping score. I was letting go of that. When I came back [from getting bagels], I could really be with her. I found that I could take care of the person taking care of Miriam. I had found something I could do. I realized that Linda was not going to do it all. I had to let go of my fear of being left out, of not being able to do it all."

Added Miriam, "He was the fresh team of horses to be brought in." Miriam had the impression that she was humming through contractions in the shower, but Tim said she was screaming through them. "I rubbed my head against the linoleum," said Miriam. "From the time they broke my water, the contractions were worse."

Four hours after being given Nubain, Miriam felt the drug wear off and was able to leave the shower. She was "glad to be back," she said. "But I was too tired, too wiped out, to continue. We had to do something." There was some confusion about whether Miriam had dilated to six or seven centimeters. When Miriam heard she might be at six, she was "devastated. I kept on waiting for transition."

Miriam was having trouble getting comfortable. Sitting was difficult and lying down was impossible. Contractions came fairly often. Finally, one of the nurses, who knew how long Miriam had been in labor, suggested an epidural.

The thought made Miriam nervous. After all, she had never thought she'd need one. The doctor came in and told them about their options. Miriam recalled that she and Tim didn't ask too many questions because they both knew they needed to do this. Together, they decided that Miriam would get both an epidural and Pitocin.

Now, the big concern was how soon she could have the drug. The staff moved quickly though. Immediately, they wheeled in the equipment needed—heart rate monitor, fetal monitor, and IV—and hooked Miriam up.

The doctor talked through what he was doing, setting up the epidural. "My biggest fear was the contractions getting worse," said Miriam. "There were needles in me, and I was shaking." The doctor laid out his instruments and went to work. "He was talking his way through it and going fast. He had a jovial voice that took the edge off the situation," said Tim.

The doctor didn't have a problem with Miriam shaking and didn't tell her to stay still. She would feel a series of little stings. Miriam, who hadn't really been listening to the doctor's description of the anesthesia, was glad that she didn't know much about it. "I didn't understand what an epidural was. It was painful. That's what it was. When I saw the epidural needle, it was a case of ignorance is bliss."

Miriam began to feel numb in a few minutes. They were assured that the amount of the drug could be monitored. Miriam would get some rest and then be able to squat, if she wanted. The doctor also cautioned them that if these interventions didn't help, Miriam might have to have a C-section. Everyone involved knew she'd been in labor for over 40 hours.

It was about 11 P.M., and Miriam felt sleepy. "I didn't sleep well though because the nurses were chatty," she said. Still, she was able to get some rest. By 1:30 A.M., Miriam was dilated to eight centimeters. The doctor instructed Tim and Linda to hold Miriam's legs. But, because of the anesthesia, Miriam had no motor control over her legs. She couldn't move. The doctor instructed the anesthesiologist to turn down the dosage. Miriam went back to sleep.

At 3:30 A.M., she woke up and felt contractions again. Now she was at 10 centimeters. "The contractions felt different, like having a bowel movement," she said.

The nurse set up the birthing bed for pushing and helped position Miriam at the end. The doctor was called in to start the perineum massage and wasn't pleased because Miriam had already started to push. "We were already seeing the head," said Miriam. "The contractions weren't devastating at this point, but the pushing took a lot. They propped me up and tried another position. This time, I was laying on my back with Linda and Tim holding my legs. I could watch as I pushed. My eyes were closed during contractions and then I watched in between. It was just great. It was a beautiful birth."

The baby's head came out farther and farther with each push. Then the head was out in two pushes. The cord was around the baby's neck. Tim was shown how to pull the baby's head out at a 45-degree angle. The doctor cut the cord. "When her head was coming out, I wasn't suppose to push very hard," said Miriam. "But then I had to push hard again, and I think that's when I tore—after the head came out. The tear was deep, but not long."

Miriam had started pushing at about 4:10 and Nina was born at 5:00 A.M. on January 12. "I pulled her out by the head and put my hands around her body," said Tim. "She looked like a cooked Peruvian potato. Not very warm, but soft. I moved her over to Miriam. As I moved her, her arm moved." That's when Tim realized that the baby was no longer inside Miriam, but a real creature, in the world. "The baby cried, and I cried," said Tim. "I was undone by it. It really touched something. At first, she wasn't the same presence I'd been associating with in Miriam's belly. But when I felt her bony butt, I could tell it was the same person."

It had been 52 hours since the start of Miriam's labor. Miriam felt pretty good now. When Tim put Nina on her chest, Miriam remembered the time she'd worked on a hog farm and helped to birth baby pigs. "A lot of the time they'd be born and get pushed onto the floor," said Miriam. "You'd pick them up and try to get them used to life. I flashed on that. We are all animals. Giving birth felt organic and very animal. And that was neat. Here was a lifeless thing, cool turning to warm. Nina was beautiful. That took me by surprise. She didn't look like I felt. She looked like a C-section baby because her skin wasn't wrinkled. I had the feeling she'd had no stress being born."

After a little while, the baby was taken away. (Miriam thought she was taken away too soon.) Tim and Carol went with the baby, while Miriam was stitched up. Miriam bled a lot afterward. The doctor looked over the placenta to find out what had happened and if the placenta had started to detach prematurely. Still, no one knew what had caused the bleeding.

The hospital had an early discharge policy, and Tim and Miriam felt that Miriam would get more rest at home. They went home at 5 P.M., 12 hours after Nina was born.

"I wouldn't have done any part of the birth differently," said Miriam. "The birth showed me what my limits were. It is possible to turn a situation around that's out of my control, but that can be better handled by other people. Having an epidural was hard for me. I usually take things as far as I can. It's hard for me to say I need help. The birth itself was so beautiful, her coming out was so incredible. That's what made it incredibly positive. If I had had to have a C-section or if she was in distress, it would have been a different story."

As for having a long, hard labor? Miriam said, "Well, that's life. My life has been like that—hard and painful. Nina's birth mirrors my experience, and that's okay. As in my life, there was this beautiful thing that happened at the end of the pain. I really appreciated that."

❦ 8

SUSAN'S STORY

RELIEF FROM NERVES

Different drugs work for different people. Susan Bjornson didn't lose her mind on Demerol, but instead got a grip on her labor. Although she had hoped to have a completely natural childbirth, she believes the drug allowed her to relax, rest, and resume labor—avoiding a C-section.

Like many other women, Susan Bjornson of Oak Park, Illinois, hoped to have natural childbirth. There seemed to be no reason why she shouldn't—she was 31, healthy, and had a comfortable, uncomplicated pregnancy.

Susan had always wanted to be a mother. She and her husband Howard weren't trying to get pregnant two years after their marriage, but that's what happened. The blood drained from Howard's face when she told him; he was shocked. "It's a scary thing, becoming a parent," said Susan.

For a caregiver, Susan chose a family practitioner. She'd wanted a female caregiver—one who had children and understood the experience of giving birth. "From what I had been reading," Susan explained, "the instance of having a C-section was less with a family practitioner." Susan didn't know of any midwives in her area and knew she wanted to have her child in a hospital. (Although she says that if she were pregnant now, she'd consider a home birth.)

Her due date was October 28. A week later, she woke up in the morning, went to urinate in the bathroom, and found blood on her toilet paper. "At first, I thought it was my period," Susan recalled. She also noticed a little wetness, possibly the leaking of amniotic fluid. When she called the doctor, she was told to labor at home and come to the hospital later that evening for a nonstress test to make sure the baby was all right. For about three hours that day, Susan walked around town with a friend. "Walking helped get my labor started. It was a positive thing for me to do. It really seemed to help keep my labor going. I didn't want it to stop." The only thing Susan didn't know was that she would be awake all night and into the next day.

At 7 that evening, Susan went to the hospital for the nonstress test. The doctor confirmed that she was definitely in labor, but not dilated, and that the baby was doing fine. It was also determined that Susan had leaked amniotic fluid that morning and had continued to leak a little all day. She was sent home and told to call her doctor if contractions became closer or increased in intensity. Susan spent that evening and night in labor. She tried to sleep but couldn't. Instead, she encouraged Howard to sleep. She continued to walk around because it was more comfortable for her. She drank a lot of water and reread books about childbirth to prepare.

The next morning, Susan and her husband went back to the hospital. They did another nonstress test and determined that the contractions were effective, even though Susan wasn't dilated. The doctor could feel that the baby's head wasn't engaged. For the first time, there was bewilderment about what was going on. Why wasn't Susan dilating?

Before the doctor could suggest any kind of intervention, Susan asked if she could continue to labor on her own. Her water had begun to leak 20 hours earlier, so there were still 4 hours before the 24-hour point. (Some doctors believe that, because of the chance of infection, labor must occur within 24 hours of membranes rupturing.)

Susan and Howard were brought to a hospital room where she could labor. The hospital had no birthing rooms, but Susan was given a room reserved for low-risk labors. She remembers the room was unattractive, with bright yellow walls. Her husband had brought videos for them to watch in the hospital. "He had brought 'Fawlty Towers,' " said Susan. "He thought for sure it would make me laugh. He had brought pictures of my cat. He was very good. But all I wanted were ice chips."

Susan continued to walk, both in the room and out in the hall. She had gone to Lamaze classes and took the instruction seriously. Susan tried to breathe the way she'd been taught, but she began to hyperventilate. "Part of Lamaze is learning how to breathe out in a controlled way," said Susan. "You don't blow a candle out; you blow and make a 'hah' sound. But I was taking in too much oxygen. My hands began to feel paralyzed and swelled up." (These are common symptoms of hyperventilating.)

Susan's labor started to take a turn. "It was awful to hyperventilate," she said. "It carried over through the rest of labor and made me uncomfortable." During this time, Susan was having contractions that appeared strong, but she still hadn't dilated at all.

Finally, the doctor gave her some Demerol so she could rest and an IV of Pitocin to see if labor would pick up. "All this made me much more comfortable," said Susan. With the Demerol, Susan didn't lose awareness of where she was or what she was doing. It even enabled her to sleep for a little while. "When the hour was up, I had dilated to one centimeter," she said.

Because she was dilating, the doctor could examine her and was able to feel the sac of amniotic fluid. The sac had resealed; the water was in the birth canal, and there was no way for the baby to get out. So the doctor broke the amniotic sac. That made the contractions come harder, and labor began to pick right up. "I was relieved that something was happening," Susan said. "There was a better chance that I wasn't going to have a C-section."

The next six hours were painful, but productive. At one point, Susan asked for more Demerol for the pain, but the doctor said no, because the baby was about to come. Susan walked around and also tried a variety of positions, including on her hands and knees. She ultimately delivered sitting back in a birthing bed, with nurses and a doctor holding her legs. And six hours after being given Demerol, Susan gave birth to her son Max, weighing 8 pounds 8 ounces. "If I hadn't had Demerol, which made me relax, I might have had a C-section," said Susan. "I attribute the Demerol to helping me avoid it."

When she became pregnant with her daughter three years later, Susan took Lamaze classes again. That time, she was careful to listen to the way breathing was described. "I wanted to really listen and figure out how to do it right. I practiced it this time," she said. During her second birth, she had more control over the pain and used no painkillers.

9

TAL'S STORY

AN EPIDURAL IN A PLEASANT SETTING

Tal Recanati wanted to give birth in a place where she felt taken care of and safe. She also knew she'd want an epidural to help her cope wth the pain. Tal, who was living in London at the time, found the perfect hospital for her birth.

When Tal Recanati was pregnant, she knew where she wanted to give birth: the Portland Hospital for Women and Children in London, England. "It's a famous [private] hospital in London," said Tal. "I knew people who had had children at this hospital, and everyone said if you're having a baby in London, you have to have it at the Portland." Tal visited other hospitals just to find out what was available. "Everyone at the Portland was nostalgic for it and missed it afterward. If you can afford it, it's the place to have a baby." (The Portland is more expensive than other hospitals in London, but comparable to or less expensive than hospitals in the United States.)

Tal and her husband, Ariel, both Israeli-Americans, had been living in London for about three years. Ariel worked in shipping, and Tal was going to law school at University College in London. Tal had an "incredible" pregnancy. "I wasn't sick for a minute. I ate and ate and had a great pregnancy. I could do it {be pregnant} every other day if it was like that."

At first, Tal's obstetrician wanted her to give birth at his hospital, St. Mary's. "He tried to convince me because that's where he felt most comfortable," she said. "But I wanted the Portland, and he knew he could deliver me there."

In England, about 70 percent of all births are conducted by midwives. It's not as common to have an obstetrician deliver the baby as it is in the United States. The Portland is an exception; many women, like Tal, have their own doctors come there.

Tal's due date, October 5, came and went. When she was 10 days late, she and her doctor decided to induce labor. "Everything was very organized," said Tal. "I had had enough. I didn't want to wait anymore. He said he would induce me anyway after two weeks. I was getting a bit tired. I wanted to be done with it. I wasn't anxious about the birth. But I couldn't wait anymore. I know some women who are into natural childbirth, and they don't want to be induced. But I wasn't so strict about those things. I was happy."

Tal wasn't anxious about giving birth and had a pretty good idea that she'd want an epidural. "I had no fear of the actual process of giving birth or having discomfort," said Tal. "I wasn't afraid of the needles or the epidural. I had a low pain threshold. I knew I would have an epidural." She had heard about a mobile epidural, which decreases the pain, but doesn't numb the body. "I looked into the epidural and decided. There didn't seem to be much of a downside or much effect on the baby. I'm not a hero. I decided that it was practical and would improve the experience if I had an epidural. That's how I went into it."

The night before the induction, Tal and Ariel went out for the evening. "We knew we were going in the next day," said Tal. "We had a good meal, saw a movie, and had a great time. We were excited."

When they arrived at the Portland the next day, it was "like checking into a hotel," Tal recalled. "It was luxurious. It has a very small maternity ward and doesn't seem like a hospital. You feel like you're at home or in someone else's home." Ariel had arranged for a suite, so Tal and Ariel had two rooms. "The rooms were wallpapered, and there was a bedroom and a living room, sort of. It was very pleasant. There was a TV in each room, a rocking chair glider in mine, and two bathrooms."

Tal and Ariel put their bags down in their rooms, and a midwife came in to see them. "She asked us some questions and got a family history." That afternoon, Tal and Ariel went out and bought candy. Their mothers came to the hospital to visit. A 7 P.M., the doctor came in to start the induction by putting a suppository into Tal's vagina.

At about 11 that evening, Tal started to feel some contractions, and her water broke. Tal and Ariel spent some time walking around. "I decided to try to go to sleep and get some rest, and we'd see what happened," said Tal. By 2 A.M., the contractions were stronger. "I called in the midwives. They took me down to a birthing room." While Ariel slept, Tal went downstairs and picked out a birthing room—she could have her choice because none was in use.

When the contractions got worse, the midwife asked if Tal would like to see the anesthesiologist. "He came and gave me an epidural," Tal said. "They attached me to a monitor to see the baby's heart rate. They wanted me to sleep. With the epidural, I didn't feel the pain very much."

Tal wanted to lie on her side, but the monitor didn't pick up very well on that side. "I had an incredible midwife at that point in the night," said Tal. "She didn't leave me for three or four hours, and kept her hand on my side so she could feel it."

At about 7 A.M., Ariel woke up and joined Tal. "The induction wasn't going well," said Tal. "I wasn't dilated enough.

The anesthesia was making me feel nauseous, so I was throwing up a lot."

There were moments when Tal couldn't decide what was worse—the pain of labor, when the anesthesia wore off, or feeling nauseous when receiving more anesthesia every hour. While Tal labored through the morning, she was joined by her mother and mother-in-law. "They were distressed that it wasn't progressing," she said. "I wasn't frightened or upset. But my mother was having a hard time seeing me, her child, in pain. Actually I was in good spirits. Ariel was wonderful."

Tal's doctor had an excellent reputation. "I would have had a cesarean in the States. He didn't give C-sections regularly." (Generally, C-section rates in England are lower than in the United States.)

Because Tal's labor was progressing so slowly, the doctor said he might try vacuum extraction, a fairly new technique in which a plastic or metal cup is placed on the baby's head and suction is used to lead the baby's head through the birth canal. "If this didn't work, he'd give me a C-section," Tal said.

First, Tal was given Pitocin. "It helped a bit, and then there was a regression. During the process, I think I actually went from seven centimeters to five. The regression was after the Pitocin."

Tal had a lot of contractions, but she wasn't dilating further. "I was lying there, hoping that it would happen soon. And it didn't. I kept waiting though. I still remember it as exciting, not as painful or awful."

The midwives, three of them in particular, were wonderful. "They had to write down every single movement, every problem, for insurance purposes. They sat and filled their notebooks. Talking and writing, talking and writing. They made suggestions. They tried to help as much as they could." Still, Tal thought the midwives felt limited by the doctor, that they had to follow his instructions. "I have a feeling when it's just a midwife, they are more in charge. But he was in charge, telling them what he wanted done and what not done. He was in and out. He came in every few hours. After eight that evening, he walked in in a tuxedo and said to me nicely that he'd see me in four hours. He was going out to dinner. That was a very British experience, having the doctor arrive in a tuxedo."

The midwives were sympathetic to Tal. She'd been the first one in the birthing room early that morning, but she was the last one out. At 11:30 P.M., the doctor came back from dinner. "He looked a little worried," said Tal. "I thought there had been some progress. They cleared the mothers from the room. He said he was going to use the vacuum to try to get the baby out. I had to push her out to a certain extent so he could attach the cone-shape that went on the baby's head. I didn't feel the need to push because of the epidural. Ariel watched the monitor and saw the contraction coming, and he'd say to push and I would. I did not feel the contractions. The baby—a girl—was born at 12:35 A.M." There was a pediatrician in the room who checked the baby, and then the midwives helped Tal nurse Danielle.

"I can't remember it, but when I pushed, the doctor cut me and did an episiotomy," said Tal. "The most surreal part afterward was when the doctor sewed me up like a tailor. He did a fabulous job because I had no pain afterward. The next day, I was up walking. I was told that he was good at cutting and repairing."

Tal spent five days recovering at the Portland. She could have the baby with her whenever she wanted, or she could rest while the baby was taken care of in the nursery. The first night, the midwives wanted Tal to sleep, and the baby spent the night in the nursery. The next five days were, said Tal, "a learning process. They taught me how to breast-feed and checked to make sure I was doing it right. They showed me how to take care of the baby—everything a new mother needs to know. A physiotherapist came in and did exercises with me for the stomach to get back in shape. You just don't want to go home. You could order the food you wanted, and they had good food."

Ariel was also able to stay with Tal and Danielle for five days. "Staying there was a nice transitional period. We were able to get comfortable with the baby in a sheltered environment before going home and fending for ourselves. That was invaluable. I understand it was a big luxury. But my five days there were probably cheaper than two days in an American hospital, and that included the doctor and everything."

In England, it's a tradition that midwives visit new mothers at home. Previously, midwives visited new mothers every day for two weeks. But because of recent cuts in funding, the midwives came to Tal less often—she had a midwife visit her every three days. "They check you and check the baby," Tal said. "They see if the breast-feeding is going all right. They were terrific." After the first few months, a community health visitor came to check that mother and baby continued to do well.

"Giving birth at the Portland was terrific," said Tal. "It provided a lovely atmosphere for having a baby. I think that I was calm and relaxed because of the setting. It helped me to feel that way. It was such a lovely place to have a child. I look back and have good memories. I don't have memories of a crowded maternity ward and no one coming to help. I really felt like an individual. I am extremely happy I gave birth there, and I'd do it again next time, if I could."

❦ 10

VICKI'S STORY

A PLANNED EPIDURAL

Vicki Placha knew that she didn't have a high tolerance for pain, and thought she'd want a drug during labor. With an epidural, she was able to experience and enjoy the birth.

When Vicki Placha of Parker, Colorado, became pregnant, she did a lot of reading and talked to many women about their labors. "You hear horror stories about natural childbirth and how painful it is," she said. "What I liked about having an epidural was that you weren't knocked out completely."

Vicki, who lived in Utah when she was pregnant, chose a local obstetrician in Salt Lake City. The doctor was a woman just out of medical school and starting her own all-female practice. "I was one of their first patients," she recalled. "Soon afterward, women couldn't get in there. They became really popular." Vicki attributed their popularity to the fact that the doctors were all women. Her doctor was also dedicated and cared a lot about her patients. "She asked me if I wanted her to be there when my baby was born," said Vicki. "I wanted her to be there. And she came in at 3 A.M. to deliver him. She knew it made a difference."

The doctor had a low cesarean rate and tended toward natural childbirth. But during early prenatal visits, Vicki told her that she wanted an epidural. "She said, 'Wait until you get to the hospital. But if that's what you wish, it's not a problem.' She didn't steer me away from it."

Vicki had an easy pregnancy. The only minor incident occurred when she was seven months pregnant. She was at work, auditing a bank. She fell down four steps on a narrow staircase in the bank. "I was concerned and called my doctor," said Vicki. "We talked for a while, and she thought everything was all right. The baby has a lot of padding then."

Vicki's labor started right near her due date. She left her job on a Thursday, and her labor started the next day. "It was like clockwork," she said. "I spent the day in labor, and it wasn't bad. I went to the doctor at 5 P.M. I had pretty good contractions then. When they hit, they hit hard. But they were far apart. The doctor told me to go home, get my things, and go to the hospital by seven o'clock."

Vicki's contractions got progressively stronger. "At home, I took a shower," she said. "I thought I'd get it done. But I began to feel as though I might not get out of the shower. Maybe I shouldn't even have come home. The contractions made me throw up. People react to pain differently. I was soon on my hands and knees on the floor. They [the contractions] hurt so much."

On the way to the hospital with her husband, Vicki lay on the backseat of the car. "The pain was bad enough when we walked into the hospital," she said, noting that she was probably dilated to five centimeters. "By the time I got there, I was ready for an epidural. They had it ready as soon as I came in and was admitted. My doctor must have told them.

"I was awake the whole time," Vicki continued. "It made it much nicer. I could feel the pressure of the contractions, feel them coming, and then watch them peak on the monitor. There was no pain."

Vicki also remembered points she'd learned in her Lamaze class—mainly about her rights as a patient. "They told us that we had a right to say who was in the room," she said. "As soon as they give you their hospital clothes, you may feel like you've lost your dignity. But you haven't lost your rights. There was a resident who wanted to come in; he needed to get his rotation in. I was almost intimidated. I would have let this guy run in, but the nurse brought it to my attention that I didn't have to. I had a choice. I believe in speaking up for what you want, and I told him no. The nurses should get more credit. In the hospital where I was, the nurses were right there with me. They were there for all the hours before the birth. They were compassionate and on the ball."

One of Vicki's most pleasant memories of the birth was sitting in the room, listening to music on her Walkman, and looking out the window at Salt Lake City. "It was a beautiful view," she said. "It was a calm moment. I sent my husband to get some food for himself. I was alone. I knew what was happening, but it wasn't painful. That had been my philosophy. I enjoyed the birth and was awake for it. I felt some of the pain of labor but have very good memories."

At one point during the evening, the doctor's partner came in and broke Vicki's water. Soon after that she had to push, and did so for an hour and a half. Her doctor came in at about 3 A.M. "We thought the baby was out further than he was," she said, "and they gave me a little more epidural [anesthesia]. It was harder to feel, harder to center, and focus on the feeling." Vicki now thinks that the extra epidural delayed the birth by about an hour.

Ty was born at 4 A.M. "I liked that I was awake and aware," said Vicki. "I was able to experience it, and my child didn't show any side effects [from the drug]. Whenever I talk to people, I explain what a great time my birth was," she said. "Women of our mother's age were cheated of this experience. There's nothing in my life that has come close to giving birth. It tops the list. Everything in life pales when you give birth.

Nothing else is the same. The birth experience was a beautiful time."

Vicki's second son, Travis, was born two years after Ty. Again, Vicki chose an epidural and appreciated her birth experience.

PART THREE

C-Section Births: Making the Best Choice for Your Baby

🌿 11

MEGAN'S STORY

WHEN LABOR THREATENS A BIG BABY

Megan Howard dealt positively with each obstacle that was thrown in her way: first, an unusual umbilical cord, then a huge baby, then a cesarean and a reaction to the drugs she'd been given. But, throughout the experience, Megan never lost sight of the fact that she was doing what was best for her child—and that a cesarean was a birth with dignity.

Five years after they were married, Megan Howard and Bruce Fretts of Hoboken, New Jersey, wanted to start a family. Megan, a managing editor for an Internet web site, found that her pregnancy went well—that is, until week 18, when a sonogram showed that the umbilical cord had only one artery and a vein. (Most umbilical cords have two arteries and a vein.) "They did a cross section of the umbilical cord and could see how many vessels were running through it," said Megan.

This kind of umbilical cord occurs in about 1 percent of pregnancies and as a result about 30 percent of those infants have some kind of birth defect, especially of the circulatory system. Because the role of the umbilical cord is to bring nutrients (such as iron and calcium) to the fetus and to take away waste products (such as carbon dioxide), a caregiver will want to make sure that the umbilical cord, although unusual, is still functioning properly.

Megan was not discouraged by this news. "I was convinced that everything was fine. I was just optimistic," she said. "They said that by eighteen weeks, if they didn't discover something wrong [because of the umbilical cord], it was unlikely that anything else would turn up."

Megan's sisters had used midwives for their births. Before she became pregnant, Megan, who was 30 years old, had been going to midwives for gynecological care. (Yes, midwives also do gynecological checkups.) "I had been going to midwives because I liked their care," she said. "My sister had told me that they were nurturing, and they were. I had been to the hospital [when one of my sisters was in labor] and saw the midwife in action. I knew that's what I wanted."

As the due date got closer, Megan, who found out she was having a boy, became aware of something else that was different about her pregnancy. She seemed to be carrying a huge baby. "I was in a birthing class with a woman who was having twins," Megan explained. "Her due date was a month after mine. People were commenting [because I was even bigger than she was]." Megan, who is 5 feet 5 inches tall, knew that big babies ran in her family, whereas they didn't in Bruce's family.

At that point, there wasn't concern about the umbilical cord. Several sonograms had revealed that the baby was doing fine. But then the sonograms began revealing the size of the baby. A few days before her due date of April 22, Megan had a sonogram, and the baby's weight was estimated at 10 pounds. The doctor (who works as a backup for the midwives and helps out in high-risk cases) called the midwives to discuss the situation with them. Megan found out the details later at the midwife's office. "I didn't understand the implication," said Megan about the baby's weight. "I thought they might induce. Then my midwife told me the gravity of the situation. The problem was that if the baby's head came down past the pelvic bone, the shoulders could get stuck. He could get stuck [in the birth canal]."

The midwife told Megan about her options. She could elect to have a C-section or wait and go into labor and see what happened. The midwife told her about what they would try if the baby did get stuck. Megan could try laboring on her side which might help get the shoulders out. Another option was to "screw" the baby out, turning him. Yet another option was to break his clavical bone (shoulder blade). Or they could push the baby back inside and do a C-section. "I spent hours crying about this option," said Megan. "I wanted it to be my decision at that point. The midwife asked me what I wanted, and I said to labor."

But Megan went home and thought about it. She really wanted to go into labor. She wanted to know what it felt like and also thought it was best for the baby. The next day, April 19, she called the midwife's office to get more information. This time she spoke to a different midwife in the practice. "I said, 'I want you to be honest. What is the worst-case scenario?' I thought it was breaking the bone. She hesitated, then said that the baby could die. There was certainly a possibility that the baby was not ten pounds and would have slid out of me. The midwife had seen these cases. But there were also others that she knew of when the baby gets stuck and can't get out and dies. I hung up the phone and said to Bruce, 'I'm having a C-section.' "

Megan made her decision right then and there. As it turned out, Bruce had been thinking that way all along. Megan decided not to wait until labor began but to schedule the C-section. "What was the point of going into labor once I knew what could happen if I labored," she said. "I also knew that he (the baby) would get bigger. If I labored and he got to that point and there were complications, it would be horrible. Why do it? Once I understood the scenario in my mind, there was no question."

Megan called the midwife's office back and told them her decision. They called their backup obstetrician. "He called me back," said Megan. "It was very nice. He just said, 'It's a big baby.' " The midwives later told Megan that she had made the choice they all hoped she would make. "I was just glad that they didn't say anything [earlier]," said Megan. "I wanted to make this decision on my own. I owned this decision."

The C-section was scheduled for April 24. There were about five days when Megan could have gone into labor and never did. "It was peculiar to know when he was going to be born," she recalled. "I felt really at peace because I knew. I felt lucky because I knew. I knew my time alone with Bruce was ending and that we'd be a threesome. That was exciting and overwhelming. I felt lucky that I had access to this technology. If I hadn't gone for the ultrasounds [there had been about eight of them], it wouldn't have been known. His heartbeat never indicated how huge he was. They were saying eight and a half pounds. It all worked out. The umbilical cord was an issue that made it all work out."

Megan went to the hospital at around 12:30 P.M. on April 24 and was prepped for the operation. "The most bizarre part was having my arms restrained," she said. "They didn't want you to reach under the sheet. I had never heard of that." But this was juxtaposed with the warmth of the hospital staff. Cynthia, the midwife, stayed with Megan and Bruce throughout the operation. Cynthia helped them arrange to have a camera with them, although it was not usually allowed in the operating room. "I felt like I got great care. It was a wonderful feeling," said Megan. The midwife, [the] doctor, [and the] perinatal doctor were all concerned about making me comfortable. There were nice, warm people all around me, cracking jokes."

When Megan got her spinal epidural, she was terrified. She had heard a horror story about a new mother whose epidural had caused an excruciating headache. (This can be a side effect of spinal anesthesia, a regional anesthetic that is sometimes used during C-sections.) "They were explaining to me about the epidural, and they made me feel so at ease," explained Megan, who held her midwife's hand.

After receiving the spinal epidural, Megan stretched out. They dropped the sheet down over her lower body. "They started pinching and poking me with the needle, but I had no feeling. I could tell I was numb," she said. "After I got the epidural, Bruce was allowed in. He wasn't there for the spinal because they don't want the husband to gasp or make a remark that makes you jump."

When Megan was fully numb, the operation began. "I couldn't tell what they were doing," Megan said. "They said I'd feel pressure but not pain. I didn't feel cutting. The pressure I felt was when Jed came out. I felt him coming out. One of the doctors said, 'This baby wasn't coming out any other way.' " Jed was born at 2:28 P.M., weighing 10 pounds 4 ounces.

Megan heard the baby right away but couldn't see him. Bruce wanted to be with Megan, but she told him to go to the baby. "Then Bruce brought him around to see me," she recalled. She asked to be taken out of the restraints and she promised she wouldn't reach underneath the sheets. "That wasn't on my mind. I wanted to touch my baby. I couldn't hold him. But I could touch him and kiss him. It was wonderful to see Bruce holding him."

Megan explained that as wonderful as the caregivers were, it was nice to have the baby's father holding him so quickly after the birth. "Bruce put him near my face. I could touch him with my hands."

The baby was taken away for more testing. "I remember the pediatrician checking him out," said Megan. "There was chaos when he asked me if the baby could be supported by formula if medically necessary. I didn't understand why they were asking me this question now. To say 'medically neces-sary' and for me to say no. It was confusing. I said yes."

Bruce, Megan, and the baby went to recovery together. It was Megan's first opportunity to breast-feed, but Jed didn't catch on. Then Megan had a reaction to the anesthesia. "I started vomiting, dry heaving," she recalled. "They said it was a reaction to the morphine in my spine. That complicated the breast-feeding. I couldn't hold him because I wasn't sure if I would need to vomit. I would get over it and try again. But it kept happening." When Jed did get on the breast, he didn't latch properly, and he was getting hungry.

When Megan went to her own room, she continued to vomit. "They kept giving me drugs to counteract the previous drugs so I would stop vomiting, and it wasn't working," she recalled. "I kept refusing each drug. I didn't want more drugs in my body. I needed the morphine in my system for the pain, but I wanted to stop vomiting. I was exhausted and scared."

Finally, after eight hours, the vomiting subsided. Mean-while, the baby had been given some formula. Jed slept, with-out waking up to eat. "The nurses would tell us that we needed to wake him up," said Megan. "He didn't understand his hunger and that he needed to wake up. He was using a defense mechanism of sleeping and conserving energy." They got con-flicting opinions from the nurses and pediatrician about whether to let the baby sleep or to wake him up to breast-feed.

Megan, who had assumed that she'd breast-feed, felt un-educated about giving her baby formula. Because he wasn't latching on properly during the two days she was in the hospital, they continued to give him formula.

When Megan got home, she consulted a lactation special-ist who discovered that Jed was planting his tongue on the roof of his mouth instead of under the nipple so he could latch on. With help from the specialist, Megan helped Jed learn how to breast-feed—which he finally did when he was three weeks old.

Megan saw the events of the birth as a continuum: "I don't think it was because of the C-section that he didn't breast-feed properly. But as a person recovering from surgery, I couldn't just get up at any hour and feed him. To me, it was a part of the birth experience. I am proud of the fact that I did keep a positive attitude and worked through three weeks of this. We were all recovering from the surgery."

The midwives and obstetrician had warned Megan that it might take her a while to recover. "When we got the baby home, Bruce went upstairs [it was a walkup apartment] with the baby. My brother, who was there to help us come home, and I hung back [a little]. Bruce was going to come back to get me, but I was right behind them at the door. I was proud. It wasn't hard. I really tried to walk a lot in the halls in the hospital. I think that helped prepare me."

Megan believes that she "absolutely had to have this C-section." Before going into the operating room, Cynthia had told Megan not to feel bad about her decision. "Even if he had been seven pounds, I would not have regretted the decision," she said. "With the information I had, I was looking out for the best interest of my child. It was all the information I had to go on. How I had this baby became less and less important as his birth approached."

Megan also recalled the conversation she had with the midwife on April 19—the one that confirmed her decision. "The midwife said to me, 'Megan, we're midwives. We want you to have a natural birth. But having a cesarean is birthing with dignity.' And I believe that."

Megan thought about all the other women who had had good experiences with C-sections. "I see it as a different kind of birth experience, rather than the wrong one," she said. "We've been told that the perfect experience is natural childbirth. But there is no one experience, and there is no one way to birth. I think that this is what every woman has to keep in mind."

❦ 12

Sarah's Story

A Home Birth Turned C-Section

I read about this woman's childbirth experience in the letters' column of *Mothering* magazine, and knew I had to find her. Here is how she sums up what happened:

> *I had a truly wonderful birth, and it was a cesarean. My husband and I had planned a home birth and labored at home with a competent, enlightened midwife. We were the strongest, most vulnerable and hardworking we had ever been. But because of a bruised cervix and the posterior position of the baby, I went from zero to seven centimeters and back to four. After thirty hours of labor—the last six of which were spent hooked up to Pitocin in the hospital—I gratefully accepted surgery. Having labored and gone through a powerful journey together, we saw this as our ideal birth. And, as it turned out, a lifesaving experience for myself and our baby.*

There was no question in Sarah Ryan's* mind: She wanted to give birth at home. A 30-year-old aspiring actress and yoga teacher, Sarah had always been skeptical about hospitals. "I didn't trust hospitals, or western medicine, or their approach

*Names have been changed.

102

to birth. I wanted a cozy, calm, familiar place. I wanted this being to come into the world in a place that was very welcoming and peaceful."

Sarah and Chuck lived in a big city but had a cabin two hours north of the city in a little town. The cabin was at the end of a dirt road on 40 acres of land in the middle of nowhere. Sarah and Chuck had bought it the year they were married. They designed it themselves; it was small, with one large family room-living room-kitchen all on one level and a sleeping loft upstairs. Outdoors, the landscape was beautiful and wild with mountain lions and deer, hawks and eagles. "It was where our birth would be," said Sarah. "In retrospect, I had a very lofty vision of what birth would be. It was more intense than I'd imagined."

The home birth Sarah imagined would take place in the small town, not the city. "In the city, we live in an apartment. I knew I wouldn't feel free there. It's a small railroad apartment, and there are neighbors around. I wanted to be where I could wander outside." The couple was used to spending a lot of time at the cabin, throughout the fall, winter, and spring.

They began their search for midwives in the city. "In the city, it seemed as though they transported women to hospitals readily, and I didn't want that to happen," said Sarah, referring to home births there. They moved the search out to the small town. "I called the local hospital, and they had one certified nurse-midwife but didn't sanction home births," Sarah said. "I asked around. There was one midwife who didn't do home births anymore because the climate here and the hospital are hostile to home births. People are afraid they are going to get arrested, practicing medicine without a license. I called another midwife and she only did home births for friends. Finally, we found out about a midwife who lived about two hours away. She had just moved to the area from another state. She'd had a great practice there." (Lay-midwifery is illegal in

Sarah's state, but legal in the state from which the midwife had moved.)

Sarah and Chuck were undeterred by the law. They weren't nervous about the birth and felt comfortable with the midwife's background. They even considered birthing the baby themselves. That's how confident they felt. "Where does that feeling come from?" asked Sarah. "There was a lot of magic around the conception. Things happened in so guided a way that we felt 'wow.' We found this piece of land and got the house built because this soul wanted to be born here. It would be nice to feel this way about everything in life.

"Other people who had children would say, in a nervous voice, knowing our cabin was on a 10-mile dirt road, 'Where is the hospital?' " Sarah continued. "I think in retrospect, I didn't want to think about anything but a simple, straightforward birth. I had to consciously work on myself a bit and say to the baby, 'We're going to have this birth at home. You can come out in water. You can come out the way you need to.' "

Sarah and Chuck took childbirth classes near their city home. When the instructor gave them a handout about C-sections, Sarah avoided it. "I didn't look at it, or read it. It described the anesthesia, and I cried because I kept thinking, 'I don't want this to happen. I don't want this to happen.' It was frightening to me. I wouldn't touch that handout. That is the ultimate irony."

They were so convinced that they'd have a home birth that Sarah and Chuck never visited the local hospital. "We did visit the hospital on the coast because that's the one that had doctors friendly to our midwife. That one was two hours away on a winding, long mountain road. But in our small town, the midwife couldn't come with us. She could be with us as our friend, but she didn't want to expose herself [identify herself as a midwife]. We were taking a big risk. We had to believe in ourselves."

Sarah and Chuck commuted between the city and the cabin in the weeks before the birth and got it ready. They put in telephone lines and ordered a birthing kit. They moved to the cabin two weeks before the March 25 due date and made preparations for the birth: They sterilized towels (washing, drying, and packing them in new paper grocery bags taped up and stored in the oven), stocked up on juice and ice chips for Sarah, and made sure they had food for the midwife, her assistant, and Chuck.

The due date came and went. A week later, Sarah and Chuck drove to the midwife's office for a checkup. "When we said good-bye, it felt odd," said Sarah. "All three of us were thinking that the next time we saw each other, I would be in labor." On the way home, they stopped off at a pediatrician's office to interview him. "I was sitting there, and Chuck was looking at me," recalled Sarah. "He said, 'Sarah, you look really different.' He interrupted the doctor to say this. I think I looked especially radiant. I felt like I was in an altered state, a little separate from what was going on around me." On the way home, Sarah had her first contraction.

That afternoon, they took a long, rigorous hike to the top of a hillside near their home. Back at home, Sarah took a bath, with yogurt, honey, and lemon to prevent stretch marks. Chuck talked to the baby the way he had throughout the pregnancy. But this time he was coaxing the baby out. "He was saying things like, 'You've got wonderful breasts to nurse at.' I interrupted him by saying, Take your time. Come out whenever you're ready. What a great environment you're coming into.' "

Immediately after their conversation with the baby, Sarah's water broke. She was on the bed, and the bed got soaked. They got towels and called the midwife. It was midnight, and she suggested that Sarah and Chuck get some sleep. The labor might take a while to start. Sarah timed the contractions, and they were about five minutes apart. "I was prepared for a long labor," said Sarah. "Our childbirth teacher had said over and over to be prepared for a twenty-four-hour labor. We were prepared."

Sarah wanted to go back to sleep, but the contractions were too strong. Chuck slept for about an hour. Sarah sat on the toilet until three in the morning. They called the midwife again, and again she suggested they get some sleep. They waited until 7 A.M. to make the next call, when the contractions were three minutes apart, regular and one minute long. "When Chuck told her about them, she said, 'Oh my, you guys. Can you handle the birth yourself?' Chuck said yes. She was worried that she wouldn't get there."

While Sarah sat and dealt with the contractions, Chuck made last-minute preparations. Because the baby might be born during the day, he wanted to cover up the windows so the light wasn't so bright. They had rented a birthing tub, and Chuck filled it with warm water.

"We had this nice morning together, once the house was set up," said Sarah. "We knew the labor was happening. We put on some meditative music. I remember standing in the middle of the room before the midwife came, and Chuck came over and gave me a hug. I was so glad to be here on the planet doing this. It was really moving."

Sarah called a few family members and friends to let them know labor had started. "It was a sweet time," she recalled. "We were so excited, and then a contraction would come and I'd hand the phone to Chuck. I just had to stop, stand there, and breathe. Sometimes I'd lean on Chuck."

The midwife arrived at about 8 A.M., examined Sarah, and determined that she was at five centimeters. The labor was going fine, and she suggested that Sarah and Chuck go out for a walk. "I had wanted this birth to happen where I could go outside," said Sarah. "But during the labor, I didn't really care where I was. I'm glad I was where I was, but I'm not sure it was as important as it was when we were planning."

Sarah had invited two people to be at the birth—Chuck's sister Maria and a friend, John. Both of them arrived while Chuck and Sarah were outside. They walked around together. "I have no idea how the time passed," said Sarah. "I held Chuck's and John's hands. We walked over and looked at the bulb garden we had planted. It was in riotous bloom. The garden had been planted for the baby."

John left, and Sarah and Chuck continued to walk around, this time down the driveway. Sarah didn't really feel like socializing, instead she wanted to deal with the contractions. The morning passed. Most of the time, Chuck and Sarah were alone; the midwife was not really interacting with them, except to check on how Sarah's dilation was progressing.

At one point, Sarah wanted everyone out of the house, even Chuck. "This was a marvelous moment for me. I wanted to be by myself. I started yelling at the contractions, saying, 'Come on, contractions. That's nothing. Come on.' I became like a warrior, just yelling at them to get stronger. I changed the energy for myself and felt empowered." Wrapping her arms around a supporting post in the center of the room, Sarah leaned back and squatted. "I felt powerful," she said. "I had decided to take control instead of having the contractions take over me." Then Sarah asked everyone else to come back in.

Soon after that, out on the porch, she had a really strong contraction. As she had done before, she gripped a post and squatted. Not all the amniotic fluid had come out earlier when her water broke. Now it did, a huge gush. Everyone laughed at how Sarah was washing the car.

The midwife listened to the baby's heart beat and suddenly got serious. She had Sarah lie down on her left side. The heart beat had slowed. When Sarah lay down, the heart beat

107

came back up. "In retrospect, I realized that the water coming down so hard had bruised my cervix," said Sarah.

She spent the next few hours going in and out of the tub and was at seven or eight centimeters dilated. Sarah couldn't eat but sucked on frozen ice chips made of juice. The midwife urged her to keep drinking. As Sarah recalled, the "labor gets hazy for me here. I know it slowed down."

It was late afternoon, and Sarah was tired. "I wanted to be in the birthing tub, relaxing. My midwife didn't want me to be in it that much. She was afraid that that was slowing the labor down."

In the early evening. Sarah suddenly felt like dancing. Chuck put on a Middle Eastern tape with lots of drumming. "I had been awake for over twenty-four hours. I danced for half an hour. It was great, standing and really moving. The midwife and Chuck clapped for me. Chuck danced for me. Afterward, I was exhausted and had to stop. The midwife checked me, and I was back down to four centimeters. That was the low point of the labor. Up until that point, I felt empowered—I felt I could do it. I was looking at starting all over again."

The midwife gave Sarah a homeopathic remedy that caused very intense contractions. They were so close and so intense that Sarah felt she couldn't handle them. "Up until then, I had moved and breathed through them. All I could do was scream and lie there. At this point, in the back of my head, I began thinking that I may have to go to the hospital. We were all thinking it."

They tried the homeopathic remedy again, but, although the contractions were intense, Sarah didn't dilate further. The midwife also realized that Sarah's cervix had become bruised when her water broke on the porch.

"At about 11 P.M., nothing was working. I don't know who said it first, probably the midwife. We should go to the hospital. But should we go to the hospital two hours away on the winding road where they knew the midwife? Or the one in our town? There was no decision. There was no way we could get in the car for two hours. I felt really scared at that point. Here I was in labor. As far as I knew, the hospital was hostile to home births and we were going by ourselves." The midwife tried to reassure them, saying that Sarah would be put on Pitocin, and that would help. The midwife also called the hospital to say that they were coming. Sarah and Chuck said good-bye to the midwife, leaving her at the house to clean up.

Maria drove them to the hospital, and Chuck sat in the back with Sarah. "I remember holding his hand and looking out the window," she said. "With the drive and feeling nervous, the labor really slowed down."

When they arrived at the hospital, they went first to the emergency room. "This is the nightmare phase for us," said Sarah. "We were in enemy territory. In the emergency room, the doctor was nervous. He was not an obstetrician. He ushered me in, and Chuck started to come, too. He told Chuck to wait outside. Chuck said, 'I'm coming in.' And he did."

Sarah was dilated to about four or five centimeters, and the doctor called the hospital (which was a building away) and arranged for Sarah to be admitted. "We rode over in an ambulance," said Sarah. "The ride was great. The driver and his assistant were in their twenties. They were joking with me. They didn't want to deliver the baby. It was a sweet thing. I remember being comforted by them."

At the hospital, Sarah was immediately hooked up to several machines—IV, Pitocin, and an internal fetal monitor. "This was our worst-case scenario," said Sarah, "but everyone was really nice. The nurses were angels. As it turned out, the nurse with me had given birth at home and was very understanding. Even our doctor was friendly."

Later, Sarah and Chuck found out that any other doctor would have rushed them into the operating room and done a C-section. But this doctor wanted to see if Pitocin had any affect on her labor. "It was a dream come true for us," said Sarah. "We relaxed. It seemed like this was meant to happen. We had done everything, exhausted all possibilities. It had been twenty-four hours of work, and I'd been awake for thirty-six. We had done everything, and this child needed to be born in a hospital. I still felt like I had choices. I was not ready to do a C-section. I still wanted to work at it. And we could do that, and I felt very comfortable."

Although Chuck tried to warn the doctor that Sarah was sensitive to drugs, she was given a regular dose of Pitocin, and immediately had massive contractions, stronger than after the homeopathic drugs. Sarah lay down and screamed. After a while, they lessened the dosage, giving her one-ninth the regular dose.

Even hooked up to the machines, Sarah could walk around and stand by the bed if she wanted. Sarah and Chuck breathed together. "I would breathe whatever way, and Chuck would breathe with me," said Sarah. "It was important that he was focused one hundred percent with me. It was really wonderful. We worked that way for another six hours."

At about 5 A.M., the doctor examined Sarah; she was only six or seven centimeters dilated. Sarah was gradually dilating, but, at the rate she was going, it was going to take another four hours before she was fully dilated. The baby was posterior, which meant Sarah was going to have to push for several hours. She was going to be exhausted, and the doctor thought it was risky to proceed. He suggested a C-section. "Chuck and I looked at each other and burst into tears because we had done everything," said Sarah. "Five minutes later, the doctor was still standing there. He said, 'I take it that means yes.' We felt relieved and completely accepting of it. Once we got over that moment of making the decision and feeling disappointed, then we were okay. We'd do it and have the baby in an hour."

It took the team about 45 minutes to get ready. People started to come in and go out, getting Sarah ready for the operation. At one point, Chuck asked for 10 minutes alone with Sarah. "We said a prayer and talked to the baby," said Sarah. "We talked to the baby about how you could be born in water and vaginally, and about how it wasn't going to be that way. He would come out through my stomach. About how his mommy wouldn't be with him right away. I'd see him in an hour. But his dad would be there the whole time. There's a prayer that we said every day of the pregnancy. We said it every day for three years even before he was born, knowing that one day he'd be born. We said the prayer before the operation. It's hard to find the right words. Chuck and I felt connected. We were doing the right thing. We had surrendered, but it wasn't at all as though we'd had a battle. We had come on a journey, and this was the way it ended. Okay."

The operation proceeded. Sarah's lower belly was shaved. Chuck went out to get dressed in scrubs. The anesthesiologist came in and explained the procedure. Sarah would receive a spinal epidural and be awake. "They started to wheel me into the operating room to do the spinal," Sarah said. "Chuck walked in, and the doctor said he couldn't come. The decision was up to the anesthesiologist. I panicked. The scariest part to me was having the drug put in—would it be a tube or a needle? When I realized Chuck wouldn't be there with me, I turned to the nurse who had shaved me and said, 'Will you hold my hand?' She said, 'Sure.' It was amazing. This woman held my hand the whole time. Every time she had to do something else, she'd tell me, do it, and then come right back. I felt so vulnerable, but these total strangers were completely there for me."

The spinal felt strange to Sarah. "I could feel the morphine they used. It made my throat tight. It wasn't painful, but

111

wasn't comfortable. It took about fifteen minutes for me to get numb."

Chuck came in, and the operation took about five minutes. "The technology was outstanding," said Sarah. "They had to pull hard. I could feel my belly moving around. They had to wrestle to get him out, pull him. They had one doctor holding one side of the incision, and the other on the other side. One of them asked for a suction cup to get the baby out. Chuck was saying mentally, 'Don't use that.' Both doctors were still pulling. Two seconds after the doctor asked for the suction cup, the baby came sliding out." And Adam was born, weighing 8 pounds.

The baby was in a posterior position (facing down) and had a big head. Sarah, who is about 5 feet 2 inches tall and weighs 110 pounds, has narrow hips. "He couldn't fit through my hips," she said.

If she ever has another baby, Sarah would make sure she was familiar with the hospital and get to know a backup doctor. "But I'd still attempt a home birth," said Sarah. "We just ignored the possibility [of a C-section], and I would not do that again. I'd still like to see if my body could do it.

"At the cabin, we had found some animal bones. I had found a pelvic bone from a deer. We had it sitting on a rail. Early in labor, I looked at it, and it was split in half. No one had touched it. After the labor and C-section, I flashed on that. To me, it was a sign that basically this baby was not going to come out. My pelvis would have split open. I believe that without this technology, we wouldn't have made it."

❧ 13

SUSAN'S STORY

A C-SECTION WITHOUT ANESTHESIA

After three C-sections, Susan Olman felt as though she was missing something essential—connecting with the baby as soon as it was born. So, during the fourth C-section when the anesthesia didn't take, Susan didn't tell her doctors how much she could feel. The irony was that during her last C-section, she got closer to having the birth experience she had always wanted.

Susan Olman of Neptune, New Jersey, was 18 when she had her first C-section. Until then, her experience with childbirth had been the stories of friends and family, most of whom had delivered naturally, including her mother, who had had eight children. "My thoughts about birth were simple," said Susan. "You go into labor and have a lot of pain, and a lot of work, and out comes the baby. That was it. The word *C-section* was not in our vocabulary."

During her first birth at a New Jersey clinic, she was eight and a half centimeters dilated when her labor slowed down. And she remained stuck at eight and a half centimeters for four hours. Her regular doctor was away on vacation, and she had a doctor whom she was meeting for the first time. "My own doctor would have let me walk around during labor," said Susan. "Instead, this doctor said, 'You're not progressing; we'll

113

have to do a C-section.' My response was to do whatever we had to do to get this baby out."

It was the mid-1980s, and at the clinic having a C-section included the full treatment: being shaved, receiving an enema, and being strapped to a bed. Susan was medicated, but awake, during the operation. When the baby came out, she was put under completely to be stitched up. "I don't really know why they did this, and they didn't tell me they were going to do it," said Susan about the extra anesthesia. "I can barely remember seeing the face of the baby. I was mortified when I woke up because it was eight hours later, and I wanted to breast-feed."

When a nurse brought 9-pound-3-ounce Robert to Susan, she was still numb from the waist down. "The nurse said, 'Watch out, he's juicy.' I didn't know what she meant. He started to choke. It turns out a C-section baby has a lot of mucus and chokes easily. What was I going to do with this choking baby? It was not very pleasant. But he was wonderful, and I was happy to nurse him and get on with it."

Six months later, when she discovered she was pregnant again, Susan had a better idea of how she wanted to deliver. She asked the doctor if she could go into labor. His answer was guarded: She could go into labor, but he cautioned that her incision from the last C-section was less than a year old, and wasn't healed enough. (Many doctors are concerned about the rupture of a previous uterine scar: *Uterine scar interruption*, as it's called, has been found in 2 percent of patients, according to the American College of Obstetricians and Gynecologists.)

Susan and her husband scheduled a C-section. "We'd been through this before, so it wasn't a big deal," said Susan. "I woke up that day and knew I was having a baby."

Susan made it clear to her doctor that she wanted to be awake during the birth and to hold the baby as soon as possible afterward. "I told the anesthesiologist that if he gave me something that made my mind fuzzy, I would sue him. They tried to convince me to have some medication while they were stitching, but I said, 'Why do it when I'm still numb from the waist down?' " Susan got the spinal epidural she wanted but admitted that the stitching was uncomfortable. "You can feel the doctors pulling and pushing which is why most women like to have something."

Afterward, Susan felt as though she had the birth she wanted. "I used to say that Vincent was my best birth, my easiest birth," said Susan. "I went in and had the operation. There was no labor. I had more control over what I wanted. It was eleven years ago and VBACs [vaginal birth after cesarean] were unpopular."

Soon after Vincent's birth, Susan heard that a friend was planning a home birth. She asked if she could be there. "My friend took pity on me," Susan said. "I'd had two kids and had never seen a baby born, and I missed that. I wanted to see it."

After witnessing her first home birth, Susan attended eight more, the births of her sister's baby and the babies of several friends. She also read up on the subject, educating herself thoroughly about childbirth. There had been something missing in her births: the close relationship between mother and baby that occurs as soon as the baby is born. "During a home birth, you could actually see the connection between mother and baby," she said. "I had never experienced that immediate connection—to do all this work, and see the baby, and know it's mine. It's such an elating time. That's what I yearned for."

Susan had several miscarriages between baby two and baby three. But when she became pregnant with her third child, her mind was made up. She was hiring a midwife and wanted a home birth. She took good care of herself, ate well, and walked two to three miles a day. She felt sure she'd have this baby at home.

Right on schedule, Susan went into labor. The contractions started off five minutes apart. They lasted four days. On the evening of the fourth day, her water broke. "I had been up for those four days," said Susan. "Every time I had a contraction, I would wake up. They were strong." Her midwife set up an inflatable hot tub in Susan's living room. With her husband at her side, Susan labored at home until four in the morning. "I was fully dilated and pushing for three hours, but nothing was happening," said Susan. "We decided then that we had to go to the hospital."

When they got to the hospital, the doctor on call read them "the riot act"—he thought Susan had gone through the entire pregnancy without any prenatal care. "I couldn't say I was seeing a midwife," said Susan. "Lay midwives were not connected to the hospital, and we didn't want to get the midwife in trouble." Susan let the doctor yell at her about the importance of prenatal care. She was still fully dilated, and the doctor let her push for 45 more minutes. Still, nothing happened. Next, the doctor tried vacuum extraction to get the baby out, but that didn't work, either. So they scheduled a C-section. "He put me out," said Susan. "He said, 'I don't know you. It's been too long.' He wanted to get the baby out quickly. Here we go again." And so Brandon, their third child, was born.

After the birth, Susan felt as though the attempt at a home birth helped her "heal a lot of problems" she'd had with the C-sections. "I had questioned whether the other C-sections were necessary. And the fact that I'd pushed and pushed verified the fact that they were necessary. That was hopeful."

When Susan went back to the doctor to get her stitches out, he told her he thought her pelvis was misshapen. "The fact that we couldn't get the baby out was a puzzle to him," said Susan, who also asked the midwives for their opinion. They did a pelvic exam and found that her pelvis was oval, not round. "They said, 'You never know when it's going to crack open and the baby will come out.' " The midwives felt bad that

Susan hadn't had a home birth. It was rare for them not to succeed; they had a 98.2 percent home-birth success rate. Of the other 1.8 percent, only four were C-sections.

Susan still wanted a home birth. "It was so important to me to feel that baby come out," she said. "I knew all my children were mine. But the fact was that I had never felt them come out of me. If anyone had given me a baby, I would have felt like it was my own. When it comes right out of you, it's what you've been carrying for nine months. The connection is the feeling of the baby coming out. Then it's yours. It was such a strong feeling to experience the pregnancy, and then there's a missing link, a period of time that's not fulfilled. That's where number four came in."

Susan became pregnant about nine months after Brandon's birth. She was again determined to have a home birth and wanted to figure out the best way for it to work. This time, she saw the midwives and went to a prenatal clinic for care so that the staff there would know her. Again, she didn't tell the clinic about the midwives or her plans for a home birth. "If I did come in with a C-section, I wanted to have some control over it," said Susan.

Throughout the prenatal visits to the clinic, Susan fought with the doctors about what she wanted. She didn't want them to just schedule a C-section. And she didn't like the way they just assumed that, after three C-sections, she was sure to have another one. "I told them that labor was important and they said, 'Where did you get that from?' Their attitude was, 'Why would I want to put my baby through all that? It's so unnecessary.' I told them about the benefits of labor and how stressful a C-section is on a baby. A baby is warm one minute and then ripped out the next. They found out that I wasn't going to take any crap from them."

Susan had educated herself well. She and her doctor argued extensively about sonograms. "I didn't think I had to

117

have one," she said. "I refused. The doctor called me into his office, and we went around and around. But I was so educated at this point that he had no argument." Susan's battle with the doctor went something like this: She'd have a sonogram if he signed a paper saying there were no side effects to a sonogram now or 30 years from now. The doctor refused to sign, and Susan didn't have a sonogram. "There was no reason for the sonogram. He wanted to verify my dates. I knew when I got pregnant. The baby would come when it was ready. I was going to go into labor, and they did not like it all. I saw twelve different doctors there, and every one said I was out of my mind, that I'd kill myself and my baby." Susan told them about home births, and they shrugged their shoulders. They thought a home birth put the baby in jeopardy.

"Sometimes in life you have to give, so you can get," she said. "I told them all the way through that I would have a C-section, but in my heart I thought I'd have a home birth. I would go into labor and push at home. If I walked in there, it would have to be a C-section. But if I was going to have a C-section, I'd go into labor first."

The doctors scheduled a C-section, and Susan boldly said she wouldn't be there. "It was enjoyable [defying the doctors], not stressful," recalled Susan. "Because I'd prepared myself for seven years with information, I was convinced that the C-sections were unnecessary, sonograms were unnecessary. I gave them a run for their money." During one prenatal visit, she spent about 45 minutes discussing childbirth with one of the doctors. "He could tell that I was well-rooted in my beliefs and said that working in this clinic, he didn't come across many women who know anything about childbirth. He thought it was a good experience for me to discuss why I wanted what I wanted."

As she did with her past births, Susan had requirements if she were to have a C-section. She wanted regional (either spinal or epidural) anesthesia, not general, so she'd be awake and would come out of recovery quickly. She wanted to hold the baby immediately after birth and to nurse while she was being stitched up. She also wanted rooming-in (the baby staying in the hospital room with her).

Susan went into labor at about 11:30 at night, and contractions were two to five minutes apart. The midwives got there at about 1:30 A.M. Susan labored all night, and in the morning she saw her children off to school. She told them they could stay home if they wanted to, but they said they'd see her after the baby was born. (The youngest, who was about 18 months old, did stay at home.) At noon, her water broke. The contractions were intense, and Susan started pushing. "I was bearing down, pushing every minute. After about an hour of that, I asked one of the midwives to put her hand up there during a contraction."

During the pelvic exam, the midwife felt the baby pushing against the pubic bone. "I was talking to the baby and to myself," she said. " *'Get past that bone. Push past it.'* I was concentrating on pushing that bone, making it crack." At 2:30, the children came home from school. Susan saw the look on their faces—the baby wasn't coming yet. The midwives checked her again, and still the baby was pushed up against the pubic bone. "I pushed with everything, with strength I didn't know existed," said Susan. "But I saw the look on my midwife's face. It's not getting past. The baby was stuck behind the bone." Susan asked everyone to leave the room except her husband. They talked about how worried her husband and the children were. They asked one of the midwives to come back in and they discussed how, if Susan were able to push the head out, the baby's shoulder might get stuck.

"Well, then, we're not doing this anymore," said Susan. They went to the hospital. "The funniest thing was that I was ten centimeters dilated and pushing, the elevators were closed, and I couldn't get upstairs. The fire company came and got me up there. I was in intense labor and wondering if the baby was all right."

Susan's labor slowed down and she went back to being seven and a half centimeters dilated. "I was not happy," Susan said. She'd read about how labor often slows or stops when a woman travels to a hospital or is moving during labor.

Susan recognized the doctor on call at the clinic. When he examined her and found that she was seven and a half centimeters, he changed his tune about natural childbirth. "He thought I could have the baby vaginally," she said. "They thought I would have torn or hemorrhaged by then. But he didn't have a clue. I told him I'd been home pushing for three hours. That I had midwives. So I wasn't going to do this. I was going to have a C-section. Let's get on with it."

They prepped Susan for the operation and gave her a spinal epidural. "I lay on the table waiting for the anesthesia to take," she said. "The anesthesiologist pricked me on the leg with a needle, then pricked my stomach. I could still feel it. He said if I didn't get numb, he'd have to put me under completely. I said, 'you will not.' I didn't care—if I had to do it without anesthesia, I would."

According to the doctor, the hardest part of the body to anesthetize is the skin. So he used a topical Novocaine. Susan's legs and hips became numb, but not her abdomen. "I felt everything," she said. "It was very painful. I felt myself being cut with scissors."

The whole procedure took about 15 to 20 minutes and the baby was out. "They pushed down when they took the baby out and pulled from the bottom," Susan said. "That pushing down on the open wound was excruciating. But I saw her instantly. I felt the little legs come through. I saw the baby. I was crying so badly. That was my baby. No one could hand me a baby and say, 'This is your baby.' That one was mine. I felt it come out of me. It's not so much the issue of it coming out of me, but the connection, feeling the birth. I felt the whole thing. I was so happy. At that point, I didn't care about the wound. I refused to let them know how badly it hurt."

They stitched Susan up, and that was also painful. "They clean you out with a power spray," she said. "They pull your uterus. It was so painful. I told the nurse that I wanted to breast-feed. They were suctioning her and wiping her down. I was crying. My husband was crying. We wanted a girl. We were so happy."

The pain was so intense that Susan felt nauseated and began to throw up. "Sometimes when you have pain so intense it sends you into shock," she explained. "At that point, while I was throwing up, the doctor yelled at the nurse because, by throwing up, I was wrenching my stomach muscles and pulling out the stitches. The nurse said, 'I can't make her stop.' " Susan got nervous. She was still afraid that they would give her general anesthesia and put her under.

She willed herself to stop vomiting. "I told them I was fine. I wasn't going to do that again. The greatest thing was I was in control. I refused to throw up, refused to get sick. They would put me out. They could put a drug in that IV, and there was nothing I could do. I had to control myself. I focused on that baby on the table." Susan got to hold the baby for a few minutes, but couldn't nurse her because she was lying flat on the table. "This was the first time that I held any of my children immediately," said Susan, recalling that she'd held her first baby eight hours after birth; the second one, three hours later; and the third, one hour, and then not again for two or three hours.

Susan was sent to recovery and the baby to the nursery, where her husband and mother would watch over her. Susan and her husband had decided that if the baby was a girl, Susan would have a tubal ligation. The procedure was performed immediately. "Yes, go ahead. We had our girl. We were done

121

with all this. Moving on to the next chapter. I wasn't put under for that, either. I felt the ripping and the tying. I didn't want to go under because of the baby."

Susan had read horror stories about women whose anesthesia hadn't worked during C-sections and how horrified they were. "If it had been my first, I would have been scared, but it was my fourth and I knew what I was missing," she said. "Other women have the opportunity to have a VBAC and experience the connection between pregnancy and being a mother. When I felt it [her daughter's birth], I made that connection. I felt that happen, going from being pregnant to being a mother. I felt the baby come out and that was amazing. Even though it sounds like such a terrible thing to not have anesthesia [that works], you don't miss that connection. Once the baby is out and the C-section is over, the issues start. You feel this sense of emptiness. You're not whole. You feel less of a woman. I didn't think too much about not having anesthesia, and I'm real glad I didn't. The message is this: Be in control as much as you can in every kind of situation."

Susan believes that her third birth was a precursor to what happened during the fourth. "When they put me under [for birth number three], I kept coming out of it," she said. "I'd say to myself, 'Uh-uh wow, this hurts. They don't know I'm awake.' " When the operation was over, the anesthesiologist told Susan that she was the hardest person to keep under he'd ever had. "I said, 'I know, I kept waking up.' With the anesthesia not taking for the fourth birth, I think it had everything to do with how long I'd labored. Maybe the natural endorphins going through my body counteracted the anesthesia."

Although being cut open was extremely painful, Susan can't compare it with giving birth naturally because she never did. "My sister said the pain of healing from a C-section is more severe than giving birth," said Susan. "A C-section hurts— you're very sore for six weeks. You're walking and laughing carefully. When you have three other children jumping around you, it's scary. You're trying to take care of the baby and yourself." With each delivery, however, recovery got easier for Susan because she knew what to expect.

Susan knows now that she will never feel the pain of pushing a baby out, but she feels that her fourth C-section was the connection she craved. "I needed that birth to get healed and to feel whole. My prayers were answered, even though it was painful. But birth is painful, too. I don't feel like I suffered more than anyone else. We are told there is a baby inside us; sonograms tell us that a baby is in there. Who really knows?"

Now Susan says that she does know. "There is little Emily. She came out of me."

14

Val's Story

Breech!

Val Harper had been born in the elevator at the hospital. She expected giving birth to her own child would also be quick and easy. But two weeks before her due date, the baby turned over. "If natural childbirth is not wonderful for your child, then it's not wonderful for you," said Val.

Val Harper and her husband Chris live in Raymond, New Hampshire, a middle-income town in a rural community located 60 miles outside of Boston. Val is a reference librarian and associate professor at the University of New Hampshire. Chris is a science teacher at a local high school.

Val became pregnant when she was 35. She had never been pregnant before and didn't try for very long before conceiving. Val assumed that she would give birth naturally. "My mother and sisters had easy pregnancies and slapdash births," she explained. "I was born in the elevator at the hospital. My mother and sister gave birth quickly. That seemed to be the pattern in my family. I had no reason to think it would be otherwise for me. We had never had a C-section in my family. We had no reason to think it would be necessary. No medical reason.

"My health plan would have let me pick any number of practitioners," Val continued. "But I was already seeing a family practitioner who specialized in reproductive health. She had been my doctor for three years. She knew the general state of my health. I went to see her the year before about getting off the pill and getting pregnant. She was in on this from early on." Even though there were nurse-practitioners, Val saw her regular doctor during every prenatal visit. She also received guidance on diet. "My nutritional intake was watched over by a nutritionist because I put on weight quickly," she said. "It was a prenatal package."

Val had a good pregnancy. "Every prenatal visit went well. I had amniocentesis and was pleased with that. We found out we were having a girl and were delighted. Everything looked sound and that made us relieved. I had never felt better in my life."

During childbirth classes, Val had the option of taking an additional two-hour session on C-sections. "We went to it to be prepared," she said. "Our health care paid for it, so we took the opportunity. That's what happens when you have an academic background. You can't stay away from classes. I wanted to know what would happen."

As it turned out, Val left work and was on maternity leave earlier than planned. "My blood pressure was elevated, and I had to lie on my left side for two hours every day," she explained. "We were still renovating the house. I would lie on my left side and work on the molding at floor level. I obeyed doctor's orders, but I had a lot to do."

There was still no reason to believe Val would have anything but an uncomplicated labor—that is, until two weeks before the delivery. On a Thursday morning, she woke up feeling bruised. "My midsection felt battered," she said. "I didn't think much of it. I had a prenatal exam later that day. I thought I'd just wait until that time and see."

The aches Val had felt in the morning went away. But, at the exam, the doctor "frowned a lot," Val recalled. "Something was not right. The baby had been head down for most of the pregnancy. This time, the head was up. That was what all the bumping and bruising had been. At almost nine months, she had turned. There wasn't much room to do it. The doctor didn't explain why this had happened. But the baby had been active and turning around all through the pregnancy. I don't know how she could turn upside down in that little space. But I was painting, I was active. Maybe I was so active that I jolted her into being active."

The doctor scheduled Val to come to the hospital a week later to see if she, along with an obstetrician, could turn the baby around. "The doctor explained what they were trying to do," said Val. "She also explained that they might have to do an emergency C-section if something was wrong, like if the cord was around her neck.

"They tried to turn her," Val continued. "This was not fun. I thought, 'If labor is anything like this, I'll go for a C-section.' It was painful. It wasn't sharp pain, but it was uncomfortable. I was hooked up to an ultrasound machine so they could determine where her head was. The doctor had experience turning babies and had a reputation for being able to do this. I was grateful that my doctor didn't try to do what she wasn't able to do and that she turned us over to him."

Trying to turn the baby was a "good team effort," said Val. The doctor tried to move the baby from the outside. "It is as though they are trying to move your organs around," she explained. "They push the baby from within, like it's a teddy bear under a blanket. They watched the fetal heart monitor and my vital signs in case the movement induced labor. The doctor had small hands which was good because he had to get his hands under her head. He really worked to push her around. He tried to make her do a somersault, at the same time keeping an eye on the ultrasound. The reasoning was that if she had flipped once, she could do it again. After ten minutes, he didn't want to continue. There was no point in trying. Her bottom seemed to be stuck in my pelvic girdle."

Val was unhooked from the monitor and given something to eat. (She hadn't eaten yet that day in case she'd had to have an emergency C-section.) "They would not attempt a breech delivery," she said, "and wanted to schedule a C-section the next week. My ability to labor was unknown to them. They didn't know what my pattern would be. I didn't care. I only cared that she be delivered in the safest, healthiest way." The C-section was scheduled for April 7 at 7 A.M.

If she went into labor before that day, Val was to call the family practitioner, not the obstetrician. "It was neat to think that my child's birthday was set," said Val. "Most people know the birthdate after, not before. You can almost send birth announcements out ahead of time."

Val felt good during the last week of pregnancy. Because of slightly elevated blood pressure, she still had to rest for a few hours in bed. But she didn't mind. She took it easy, finishing up last-minute details at home and getting ready for the baby. One evening, she helped Chris move a few boxes upstairs. They had just finished renovating the second floor and were getting ready to sleep there. Early the next morning, Val had diarrhea and didn't think much of it. That evening, Chris made a big, heavy dinner, and they both ate well.

At 8 P.M., Val started to feel contractions. They were five minutes apart at the beginning and soon became regular. "I had had some minor contractions previously, but they hadn't been consistent," said Val. "I had dismissed those. These were not minor. I decided to take a shower, thinking that would feel good. While I was in the shower, my water broke. I thought, 'Now, we have something here.'"

Val called the family practitioner and was told to come to the hospital. It was 11 P.M. "I was excited because the C-section was not going as planned," she recalled. "I like spontaneous things. I wasn't nervous about having surgery. I had had knee surgery four times. I'm interested in health and medicine and curious about what goes on. I wished I could stay awake and see all the procedures. We went to the hospital excited. Our daughter was going to be born."

Val was aware that some women do attempt labor with babies who are breech. Even this didn't bother her; she trusted her doctors. Although she wasn't frightened of birthing a breech baby, she had a feeling it would be more difficult. "I could have fought more," she admitted. "But once they discovered they couldn't turn her, it seemed like nature hadn't designed her to go that way."

When Val and Chris arrived at the hospital, Val was hooked up to an ultrasound machine to monitor contractions. "The doctors wanted to make sure the cord wasn't around the baby's neck," said Val. "I was monitored until the operating room was ready. They gave me a catheter, checked on my well-being, and left us alone. I focused on dealing with the contractions, which were three minutes apart and gaining in strength. They never did check my cervix to see how dilated I was. I had been in labor since early that morning. The diarrhea was my body getting set up for labor. I would have liked to know. Was I going through labor as fast as my relatives? I'll never know this. There was no reason to take the time to do it."

Two hours later, at 1 A.M., the operating room was ready. Val was wheeled in and given a spinal epidural. "I became numb from the waist down," she said. "I couldn't feel a thing. The doctor who did the epidural was good. I was comfortable, excited, and alert. Both Chris and I were soaking up what was going on."

There were a lot of people in the operating room: the family practitioner, the obstetrician, the pediatrician, the anesthesiologist and his assistant. "It was a busy place," said Val. "Everyone was in good spirits. We were cracking jokes. We could have brought out some wine. It was a pleasant experience, except for the catheter."

Val felt fortunate because she had both doctors with her, the family practitioner and the obstetrician. "I'm not sure if this is routine practice, but the family doctor was involved all the way through," said Val. "It was a team effort, and I liked that. I like having that connection and continuity with her [the family practitioner]."

Although she was numb, Val could feel the doctors moving around. "I felt pressure, no pain—just fingers, the sensation that they were there. I could see them behind the cloth and see where their hands were." The cloth was up between two posts, and Val could also see the doctors' heads over it and hear their conversation. "They said, 'Here's the head. Make the incision here.'"

At one point, everyone in the room debated what time it was. "It was Easter Sunday. We had changed the clocks at 2 A.M. because of daylight saving time," said Val. "Caitlin was born at 3:03." She weighed 6 pounds 7 ounces.

As they were taking the baby out, Val's uterus ruptured vertically. "I had to be sutured internally in both directions," she said. "As they stitched me up, they told me about this problem. They said that if I had another baby, I would have another C-section.

"I didn't see the baby until they carried her to a warming bed," Val continued. "She had good lungs. Her Apgar was great. She was healthy. I could see her from where I was, but they never pointed her out to me. No one said, 'Here's your child.' No one said, 'It's a girl.' The two doctors were busy cleaning and sewing me up. The pediatrician was with the baby."

Val was wheeled to the recovery room where she fell asleep and slept until 6 A.M. "There was a nurse at the foot of the bed when I woke up. She asked how I was feeling. Could I

129

feel my toes? My hips? She checked whether the anesthesia was wearing off. An hour later, I had regained a lot of sensation and was feeling awake. My husband was waiting for me when I got to my room. The baby was in the nursery. Chris stayed with me for an hour and then went home to get some sleep.

"They brought the baby to me around nine or ten in the morning," said Val. "It was the first time I held her. It didn't bother me that it hadn't been sooner. It had been a long day, and my body had been through major surgery. I needed to rest. We had a whole life together. I would have plenty of opportunity to hold her."

Val started to nurse, and the baby took right to it. After holding the baby for a while, the nurses wanted Val to move around. "That hurt," she admitted. "I had stitches. Sitting up hurt. I knew, though, that the faster you move around, the faster you recover—and the better it is both emotionally and physically. It's also better for your spirits."

Val was hooked up to a new kind of patient-controlled pain relief. When she wanted to, she could dispense pain-relief medication by herself. "It was hard the first day and then got progressively easier," she said. "By the third day, I was in and out of bed without assistance or painkillers. By the fourth day, I was walking around the hospital for exercise and felt great."

After four days in the hospital, Val and Caitlin went home. Val was told not to climb stairs, but she felt good and climbed them anyway. With her mother-in-law there to help, Val could take care of the baby and leave the household chores to others. "I just enjoyed the baby for the first few days," said Val. "I was physically tired, but not drained." A few days later, Val was walking around the neighborhood with the baby in the carriage and felt fine. It was an "easy recovery. I had a harder time recovering from knee surgery than from the C-section."

About her experience, Val said, "It's easy to have a good attitude when everything is going all right. But I am optimistic about having a family, about birth, about taking care of myself. I'm energetic, and that seems to be a form of optimism. Sure, I would have liked someone to point to Caitlin when she was born and say, 'There she is.' I would have liked to know why my uterus ruptured. But in general the hospital took good care of me.

"For both my husband and me, the way our child was born was not important," Val continued. "We had always thought we'd have natural childbirth if we could. But we couldn't, and there was nothing wrong with that. In our childbirth class, we talked with a couple whose child had been in distress during labor and how they were still determined to have natural childbirth. We were disgusted that they might put preconceived notions of childbirth before their child's welfare. Are people proud about the possibility of their child being brain damaged—all because they want to have natural childbirth? That seemed to us to be the wrong decision. I had taken good care of myself during pregnancy so I wouldn't hurt my child. I wasn't going to take a final chance during birth.

"The purpose is not to have natural childbirth or a C-section, but to bring a baby into the world. Giving birth is just one step you take in her development. It's an eighteen-year process. This one thing was not going to ruin, or alter, her life or ours. We felt very strongly about this. We weren't upset. We weren't even disappointed. We wanted the best thing for our daughter. The birth was positive. Really, nothing could have brought me down."

❧ 15

JANE'S STORY

IT'S NICE TO KNOW WHEN

Like her mother, Jane Gerson was having a big baby. That was the first reason to consider a C-section. Then Jane's topical herpes flared. Now, there was no choice. Jane Gerson had a C-section and felt it was the best birth possible.

Jane Gerson* of New York City describes herself as someone who does worry—but relaxes—in difficult situations. This was a quality that came in handy when it was time for her to give birth. "Sometimes, there is a point at which you can do nothing," said Jane. "If you don't worry, then you allow yourself to have more strength. You're much more in the moment."

Jane, who worked in the special events department of a sports magazine, had an easy pregnancy and was extremely active. She bicycled, exercised, and kept working right up to her due date. "At nine months, I pulled off a walking event for one thousand people," she said. "I was up at 6 A.M., getting the track ready."

A week before the due date, Jane had a sonogram. "One technician did it, and he called two other technicians over," she explained. "They calibrated the weight at eleven pounds. At

---

*Names have been changed.

that point, because of the size, it became a medical risk. That's what they told me. It didn't sound good. It was not a good bit of information to get a week before. You don't want to go into labor with the deck stacked against you."

Jane had the sonogram on Friday. She had the weekend to think about it and a doctor's appointment scheduled for Monday. She talked to a lot of people. From friends, she got the message that she should go for natural childbirth. From her childbirth instructor and people she knew in the medical profession, she heard a different message: It wasn't going to be easy. "They said that, with a big baby, your chances of having a C-section are greater," said Jane. "If you try for natural, there's the possibility that the head will come out, but the shoulders—because they're so big—will get stuck. I was very uncertain." Large babies ran in Jane's family. "My mother gave birth naturally. I weighed nine pounds eleven ounces, and my sister, ten pounds five ounces," said Jane.

For the past ten years, Jane had had a chronic form of herpes. Every once in a while, maybe once or twice a year, she would get a slight rash, always on the same spot on her back. "I went to the doctor's on Monday and pointed out the patch on my back," said Jane. "Herpes is a minor thing usually, but it's a major problem when you're pregnant. They want you to have two weeks clear of herpes before they'll let you give birth naturally. The decision to have a C-section became a no-brainer—which was nice. There was no decision to make. Now we had to have one." (If a pregnant woman is infected with herpes simplex virus, the baby could catch it passing through the birth canal. If contracted, the disease could cause death or blindness in a newborn.)

The doctor scheduled Jane for a C-section a week later, on her due date. "We went out for a family dinner the night before the birth," said Jane. "It was my mother-in-law's birthday, an elegant dinner and a special evening. There was never going to be another night in our lives like that."

133

Labor of Love

The birth was scheduled for 8 A.M. on September 30. "We [Jane and her husband Jack] walked down the street at 6:30 A.M.," she said. "It was a late summer day. We were peaceful and calm. In retrospect, the difference between a planned and unplanned birth is you don't have to do the work beforehand in a planned birth. You are not exhausted."

During childbirth classes, Jane was instructed to bring an object that she liked to the hospital, to focus on during the birth. She had chosen a small painting. "Everyone was humoring me about it because I wasn't going to be looking at a painting during a C-section," she said. "I didn't know what to expect, and brought it anyway."

When she was prepared for the operation, Jane was nervous. "They tried five times to get the needle in me. The doctor said, 'If it doesn't go in this time, we'll have to do general anesthesia.' On the next try, they got it in. I didn't want general."

As it turned out, Jane was also given a drug to take the edge off her nervousness. "When they opened me up, they put pressure on my stomach," said Jane. "Two people pushed on me. That was shocking. It was frightening to have your stomach opened up. I was shaking. It was probably a good idea to calm me down. It took the edge of recognition or remembering off. I was in an altered state. I didn't care all that much. I looked at the baby when she came out. I remember feeling good because she was there, and then wanting to close my eyes and sleep. I must have because I don't remember anything for a while."

Healing wasn't difficult for Jane. "It was a fast recovery. But the first day you can't do anything. When I finally got up and had Charlotte in my arms and started to nurse her, everything was back to normal. By the end of the first day, I was thinking clearly. I remember that fondly."

Jane had no negative feelings about her birth experience. "The focus of my pregnancy had been to have a healthy baby,"

134

she said. "As a cesarean, it was the best it could be. What took the place of it immediately was the joy of having a baby. When the birth was over, it was over. The whole point was to have a child, and here I had a wonderful one."

A few years after Charlotte's birth, Jane had an ectopic pregnancy, a pregnancy that occurs outside of the uterus, commonly in a fallopian tube or in the peritoneal cavity; it can cause death and is most always considered a medical emergency; most caregivers want to remove the embryo before rupture occurs). They were at their country house and Jane felt slightly crampy, as though she had gas. Her stomach felt very full. "It could have been nothing, or it could have been a miscarriage," she said, noting that she and Jack had, at that point, "not stopped trying."

"I called my doctor in the city and he said, 'Promise me that you will go to the nearest emergency room.' That piece of advice saved my life. I was forty-five minutes away from an emergency room. I didn't feel that bad. But according to the sonogram, I was in crisis. There had been a lot of internal bleeding. I had blood up to my chest cavity. I was saved because the doctor had been so cautious. He scared the living daylights out of me."

The next year, Jane had a sonogram to check her condition after the ectopic pregnancy. "They thought they saw a fetus at eight weeks," she said. "When I went back again, at four months, I had a placenta progressing, but no fetus." Jane had what is called a *blighted ovum*. "I had to have a D & C [dilation and curettage]. Afterward, I didn't stop bleeding right away. There was a funny look to the placenta, and, for two days, I thought I might have cancer. The doctor took me from the clinic to the hospital to have me under observation. I had 'transference' with this doctor, the way some people do with shrinks. I remember distinctly sitting there, waiting to be taken to my hospital room. I said to him, 'It's not easy having kids.'

135

He said, 'My feeling about life is that you're skating on thin ice over a minefield.' That confirmed my feeling—that at best, pregnancy is wonderful. But at its worst, there is a lot of risk. To me, childbirth is just the means to the end."

After both of these medical emergencies, Jane just wanted a healthy pregnancy. "I wasn't going to go bonkers about having natural childbirth," she said. When she became pregnant, she stopped worrying about whether the baby was all right after the third month.

"I had a friend who was having a VBAC," Jane said. "She went three weeks past her due date. I thought that was ego-driven. Everything turned out fine. Maybe it's a question of not knowing what I missed out on. But to me, having a child is more important than the birth itself." During the second pregnancy, Jane wasn't as involved as she had been with the first. "It was fun because I had Charlotte going through it with me," said Jane. "It was fun to have a kid listening to her sister."

That summer, Jane and her family went to the country and stayed there until a week before the due date. When she returned to the city, she had a sonogram. "I was assuming it was another big baby," she said. "The second one is always bigger, they say. So I felt it would be another nonissue, another eleven- or twelve-pound baby. But it wasn't. This baby weighed about nine pounds five ounces, which was in the realm of the possible. It made me think through the whole thing. The first C-section had been a nice experience. That was what I was used to. I wasn't prepared to have a hard time."

But Jane's dilemma again faded. A week before the due date, her herpes flared. "Again, having a C-section was a nonissue," said Jane. "But I do realize that I could have gone past my due date and seen if the herpes was gone. In both pregnancies, that would have been an option. I could have tried natural childbirth after having a clear test of herpes."

Jane maintained that there was an enormous difference between her first and second C-sections. "I had learned from the first one. This time, I knew what to expect. I had an anesthesiologist who didn't believe in Demerol, so I didn't have any mood relaxants, and I remember this birth clearly. That would be my recommendation to anyone having a C-section. I felt the pull on the stomach. The doctor and nurse were pushing. It's not as though they open your stomach all the way. They make a four-inch incision and then have to get the baby out of it. They push on either side and pull her out. It's an action that you're disconnected from, and that's weird. But it's not weird if it's expected. I knew not to be scared. I was much more conscious. I heard her cry, screaming like a banshee. I spent time looking at her. I might have touched her. I remember saying to Jack, 'I'm so happy.' They took her away and gave me something. I know because, later, I woke up. In both of my births, in my absence, Jack held the babies, gave them water. He has very vivid memories of the first few minutes. I have the memory of the next ten years.

"I was thrilled, and felt unbottled gratitude," Jane continued. "My feeling about giving birth is that you're in there to have a baby, not to experience the peak moment of your life. I think it's important to go into it without having expectations that will disappoint you in the end. Everything began when my children were born."

❧ 16

KARI'S STORY

A LIFESAVING OPERATION

When Kari Garcia Fisher was seven months pregnant, she gained a lot of weight and began to feel swollen all over. Luckily, a midwife's appointment at just the right time saved her life.

"Maybe we will, maybe we won't." That's what Kari Garcia Fisher and Vladimir Garcia Gutierrez of Brooklyn, New York, thought when they considered having a baby. "We loved the idea of having a baby," said Kari. "But, looking back, maybe we should have waited. Career-wise, we were not in the best of places. But we never had a minute of not wanting a baby. It was so wonderful just to be having one."

Vlad worked in a factory and was also a writer. He also did volunteer work in the Latin community. But his hours at the factory were cut during Kari's pregnancy. Kari was 30 years old and worked as a sales associate at Williams Sonoma. "My job was getting more stressful," she noted. "It was a retail job, and there was a new manager trying to revamp things, wanting us to do research at home." Kari, who wrote fiction in her spare time, had been at the store for two years and ended up staying during her pregnancy because of the health benefits. She worked full-time, putting in 40- to 60-hour weeks.

Kari, originally from Colorado, had always wanted to have her baby with a midwife. "I had babysat for two midwives in Pueblo," she said. "I had also been involved setting up a food coop when I was twelve and met a lot of midwives. I'd done a lot of reading. It seemed to me that that was the way it was supposed to be. No one in my family had problems having children. My mother never had morning sickness. She had my sister in fifteen minutes. They were used to doctors, but they were okay with midwives."

Kari had moved to the New York City area only two years before becoming pregnant. She hadn't needed much medical care since she'd been there. "When I found out I was pregnant, I started calling doctors to get an appointment," she said. "I couldn't find a gynecologist who would see me. It was a pain in the neck. I was confused. What do people do? Make an appointment to have a baby? It was weird."

For a while, Kari even thought about having the baby at home. But then she found a midwifery service in Manhattan, near where she worked. "I went to their orientation session and knew I wanted to go with these women," said Kari. "I felt so comfortable with them. I thought I had to go to an obstetrician for the first appointment. I didn't think midwives could do it. At first, it seemed that if I went to a real doctor, it would keep Vlad's side of the family happy. He comes from a country [Nicaragua] where there isn't good medical care. So they wondered why someone was choosing not to go to the doctor."

Although Kari loved the idea of being pregnant, she was physically uncomfortable. "I had horrible morning sickness. With me, it was morning, noon, and night sickness. I felt miserable for four months. I was on my feet all day at work. I'd come home and be swollen. I had trouble eating. Everyone said, 'Eat little bits all the time.' Nothing would help. But I had to eat something. I tried crackers. That didn't help. Nothing was a safe food. I threw up all the time, three or four times a day—at work, too."

After the first four months, Kari was less sick and got some of her energy back. She was still tired. Work didn't help. "It was physically a lot to do," she said. "You think of retail as waiting on people, but you are up and down stairs, getting merchandise, cleaning and lifting blenders and food processors. Finally, at Christmas time, one of the midwives wrote a note saying I couldn't be running up and down stairs all day. My blood pressure was up, and it had never been up before in my life. My ankles and hands were swollen a bit, and my face a tiny bit puffy. We thought it was all the running around."

Kari's problems got worse. She was two months away from her due date, but there was a week in mid-January when she didn't feel well at all. "I had done something to my shoulder," said Kari. "It felt sore. I was just feeling pretty horrible. We had several blizzards, and I had to reschedule my midwife's appointment." She rescheduled it for January 18 at 11:30 A.M., and then planned to go to work afterward.

Because of the snow and how she'd been feeling, Kari hadn't been out of the house in three days. "I couldn't put my own shoes on," she said, explaining that her feet were that swollen. "I had to wear Vlad's shoes."

They arrived at the midwives' office, and it turned out Kari's appointment wasn't until 1:30. "I still felt ill," said Kari. "The receptionist said she'd squeeze me in. I went to take a urine test. (At the midwives' office, patients do their own tests.) When I compared the colors on my urine stick to the chart, they were every color of the rainbow. None matched. What do I do? They took my blood pressure. They said, 'You had better go to the hospital. Do you have cab fare?' "

The midwives suspected that Kari had preeclampsia, an illness that affects a small percentage of women late in pregnancy. (The symptoms are high blood pressure and swelling.

The cause is unknown. The treatment is often to get the baby out as soon as possible or to carefully monitor the woman's blood pressure in the hospital.) "I'd heard of it, but it wasn't ringing any bells," said Kari. "I asked if maybe I should have relaxed more. But the midwife told me that this was not in my head. It wasn't something I could control. It was a physiological problem at this point.

"As I was leaving [the office], the midwife told me that I'd either have the baby today or in two weeks. They'd admit me and keep me there under observation. They made it sound like I had some time. I think she was trying to calm me down. But I was so out of it that I didn't really realize what was going on."

Kari and Vlad went to the hospital in a cab and reported to the neonatal unit. "I walked in and introduced myself, and they knew who I was," she said. "That was the first indication that something wasn't right." They did ultrasound and other tests, checked her blood pressure, and Kari was admitted. One of the midwives, Cynthia, was on call at the hospital. She tried to help Kari make last-minute arrangements with her insurance company. (Some insurance companies like patients to give them preapproval, telling them ahead of time when they'll be going to the hospital.)

"They came in with the results of the ultrasound. There wasn't a lot of fluid around the baby. Cynthia said, 'It's still your decision, but there is some danger. We can induce labor, but there's a ninety-five percent chance that we will be doing an emergency C-section in twenty minutes.' I wasn't dilated at all. We thought about it for an instant, but it wasn't even a question. I had been my friend's labor coach when she was induced. The only thing that terrified me more than a C-section was being induced. I had to remember that the whole point was having a baby safely, not the experience itself. Vlad and I looked at each other and said, 'Of course, we'll do a C-section.'"

While the staff was getting the operating room ready, Kari tried to get her insurance company on the phone. "I was talking with the insurance company when the doctor came in and took the phone out of my hand," Kari said. "She talked to the other person and said, 'We're getting ready to deliver a baby here. This is life-threatening surgery. I can't believe you're dealing with paperwork.' "

They took Kari into the operating room. "I was out of it," she said. "They did preoperation stuff. I remember they were trying to get leads into my neck to monitor the high blood pressure. They couldn't give me much of anything to numb that. They didn't want to give anesthesia until we were closer to pulling the baby out. There were a lot of lights and a lot of people—maybe twenty or thirty in the room. They were coming in and out, putting things on different parts of my body. When I'd been a labor coach for my friend, I remember she didn't mind being naked. I thought it would be an issue for me. But who cares? Let there be forty people in the room, or fifty. It just wasn't a problem."

It took a while for the doctor to get the leads into her neck, and it was painful. (Kari still has a tiny hole in her neck from the lead, but thinks it will heal further.) "Everything happened so fast," said Kari. "They determined that my blood pressure was up over two hundred. They were rushing to get the baby out before something terrible happened. I was joking around. They told me to quit trying to make them laugh.

"They cut me open, and I was in and out of consciousness. They gave me general anesthesia so I couldn't really feel it. I woke up later. Genesis was born at 5:17 P.M. on January 18. It was also my grandmother's birthday. I was still completely swollen, my feet and hands. I was puffy like the Pillsbury doughboy."

The baby was fine, but tiny. Born six weeks before Kari's due date, she weighed 3 pounds 5.8 ounces. "They had her on oxygen for a day," said Kari. "For a few weeks, she had to be fed through a plastic tube down her mouth. She made a lot of progress. They took her off the oxygen and just had her on monitors."

Kari was put on medication for high blood pressure. It took a while for her to recover and for the swelling to go down. "It was three days before I could see her," said Kari. "I was so sick. I had a catheter, IV, the whole nine yards. I was pretty out of it. Finally they took me down to see her in a wheelchair. I was able to hold her. Sometimes I think about missing her first cry. But it was the most profound thing to hold her when she was three days old. Before this, I'd thought, if you had a C-section, it wasn't a real birth. Then all these things happened that I hadn't even considered. I thought I'd have natural childbirth. I thought she'd be late and I'd be ready. It was wonderful to find out life could hand you a different kind of miracle."

Although she was still weak, Kari was able to go home after a week. The baby stayed in the hospital for almost another month. "It was sad, going home without her," said Kari. "Rationally, you tell yourself the baby needs this extra time. She's getting the best of care. But you can think about it all you want, your heart knows your baby is far away. When I was in the hospital, she was only an elevator ride away. She felt close. When I got home from the hospital, she felt a million miles away. We made the trip from Brooklyn to the hospital every day to see her."

After a few weeks of visiting Genesis, one of the nurses asked Kari if she wanted to try breast-feeding. "I said, 'Wow.' It took some doing, but she took to it pretty well."

Genesis was able to come home on February 14. She weighed 4 pounds 6 ounces. Kari was beginning to feel better. "At my six-week checkup, I'd lost sixty pounds. I had gained an enormous amount during the pregnancy, about sixty or seventy pounds. Most of it was at the end. I was getting back to the way I'd been before the pregnancy—healthy."

Despite everything that happened, Kari felt positive about the experience. "I had no idea what supportive family and friends we had. The midwives were there for everything and continued to see me, even though I was really no longer their patient. I loved the hospital staff. There were a thousand acts of kindness.

"I have no regrets about how we did it," said Kari. "It was the best of everything. It was just one of those things that happened. There was nothing I could have done differently. I was just lucky that I walked into the midwife's office on that day. My appointment had really been for 1:30 P.M. At 1:30, I was at the hospital, being prepped for a C-section."

Genesis continued to thrive. When she was two months, she weighed 8 pounds 5 ounces.

PART FOUR

Feeling Great the Next Day: Stories of VBACs (Vaginal Births after Cesarean)

🌿 17

LIZ'S STORY

DETERMINED, FLEXIBLE, AND GOING FOR IT

Liz Benson never went into labor when she delivered the first time. So she approached her second pregnancy as though she had never given birth. She knew everything about being a mother, but nothing about labor and delivery.

When Liz Benson was pregnant the first time, she had a busy schedule. She was the executive director at Settlement Health Center, a community clinic in East Harlem in New York City. Liz worked 50 hours a week and also found time to swim and exercise. A tall striking woman with blond hair, Liz had been a swimmer in college and continued to be athletic. She and her husband, Dan, lived on the Upper West Side so that they could be close to Central Park. Liz, originally from Wisconsin, could always be found running or ice skating in the park, depending on the season.

Liz felt good during her first trimester. It was summer, and she cut back her work load to 40 hours a week. She took Fridays off and enjoyed working at home. There seemed to be only one hitch in her pregnancy: The sonogram during the first trimester had revealed a fibroid the size of an orange. Because the baby seemed fine and everything else was normal, no one worried about it.

During her second trimester, Liz went back to the full-time work schedule. "I didn't know about putting limits on myself. At about this time, I remember I walked to a meeting. Usually it was a quick walk; but this time it took me twenty-five minutes to get there. I realized I had to slow down. Everyone said you can do whatever you want when you are pregnant. But my legs would get swollen by the end of the day. I ran around a lot. I figured I could. My body wasn't telling me I was tired."

But then during the second trimester, Liz had to slow down. "I started bleeding," she recalled. "It was a little like period bleeding, but different. It was enough bleeding to cause some concern. I was in my thirty-second week. We weren't sure where it was coming from."

Liz went immediately to the doctor's office so he could check the amniotic sac. "Our assumption was that the fibroid had grown and hit the amniotic sac. That was his biggest concern," said Liz, who noted that amniotic fluid wasn't leaking and that, even after the birth, no one knew what caused the bleeding.

Liz was sent home and instructed to go on bed rest. "The doctor told me that if I didn't, I'd be in the hospital." Liz was under the impression that at 35 weeks, the baby was almost full term, so it didn't really matter what happened. "But the doctor said that this was the most important time," said Liz. "The baby gains a lot each week, maybe even as much as one pound a week. I was under the impression that I was close enough. But the doctor wanted the baby to stay in for the full forty weeks.

"I remember later reading a newspaper article comparing medical residents who were pregnant versus women [residents] who stayed at home," continued Liz. "They said there was no difference in outcomes. But there was a little asterisk at the bottom of the page. It mentioned how many of the residents ended up on bed rest after working seventy-hour weeks. The outcome may be the same, but the pregnancy is certainly different."

Liz spent the first week on bed rest unwinding and taking care of business at the office—by phone. "When work at the office was done, I had a great time just chilling out. It was good. I also liked having time off before the baby. Going directly from work to the hospital—there wasn't much time to focus on the baby coming."

Liz knew that her bed rest was easy compared to other stints she had heard of. "Some women have to lie on their side," she said. "I just had to stay in bed and could get up to go to the bathroom." After four weeks, Liz was able to go out. She went to the movies, did errands. But she knew now not to overdo it and to take cabs instead of walking long distances.

Liz's due date was between Christmas and the beginning of January. Two and a half weeks into January, there was no sign of labor. The baby was still high, jutting out from under Liz's breasts, taking up the space between her belly button and rib cage. "Everyone else who is eight months pregnant complains about having to go to the bathroom a lot," said Liz, explaining that this baby never got low enough to put pressure on her bladder.

In mid-January, Liz went in for a nonstress test. "Nothing was happening," she said. "The baby was really high up. The doctor couldn't induce labor because the baby was so high, and wasn't in the birth canal. We'd get some action, but the baby wasn't there yet. We'd end up with a C-section."

A few days later, Liz was in the laundry room of her building and began to bleed again. It was a fair amount of blood, but she wasn't hemorrhaging. "At first, I was happy," Liz said. "I thought my water had broken. But it was blood." The doctor told Liz to meet him at the hospital. They checked, and the baby was fine. The doctor didn't know what had caused the bleeding, and he also didn't see any sign of labor. "He was getting concerned," said Liz. "He said, 'I'd like to do a C-section and get the baby out. Tonight's a good night.' " The doctor had no other deliveries that night, and [he had] two residents with him.

"My doctor and I had a good relationship," said Liz. "We talked things over. I could tell by the way he looked at me that he didn't want me to sit and wait. He didn't want this to turn into a real emergency. Dan and I talked for a minute. We were pushing this longer than we liked anyway. We had our discussion, and I was resigned to it [the C-section] at that point."

Liz remembered the operation fondly. Dan had brought music, and they played it during the operation. Dan had also brought an audio tape recorder to record the baby's first sounds. The anesthesiologist said he would tell Dan when the baby was coming out so he could turn the recorder on. "The doctor said, 'It will be very soon now,' " recalled Liz. "And then there was a long pause. I felt a tug of war. I couldn't feel anything below the neck. But I felt tugging going on. I heard the doctor grunting and heard him say, 'This is a really big baby.' It took him a long time. The doctor was concentrating so hard. Afterward, Dan went to the post-op meeting and found out that the fibroid was the size of a cantaloupe. The doctor had to stretch his hands around it to get the baby out. Many doctors would have cut up the other way—vertically— to get the fibroid out of the way. But then I'd have to have another C-section. The doctor wanted me to have natural childbirth if I gave birth again. They got the baby out. I saw him. Dan held him near me. And then we named him. We read the list of names, and he [the baby] stopped crying when we got to Benjamin. So that was it."

Being stitched up was unpleasant for Liz. "I got the shakes after the baby came out. That was hard for me. I got wacky. It took a while, maybe forty-five minutes. I'm not sure. I started to lose patience. There were a lot of layers and a lot of stitching. The anesthesiologist was talking to me. Dan had gone with the baby, but they told him I needed him, and he came back in. The doctor was very thorough. He was conscious of how I'd look in a bikini, even though I wasn't concerned about that."

Four years later, Liz's second pregnancy was stress free compared to her first—on purpose. She had left her job a few months before. "If I was tired, I wanted to be able to relax," she said.

This time, Liz wanted to try natural childbirth. Her doctor was supportive. "Even after the first birth, he'd said, 'Wait and see what happens.' He wanted me to have a VBAC. I was optimistic about natural childbirth. I worked toward it. For the first birth, I took Lamaze classes and wasn't particularly invested in it. I thought I'd figure it out when the time came. My mother told me that I should figure out how to relax. This time I was committed to being relaxed. I took the Bradley course and read the book, and it helped. We did the exercises from the book. We believed that having no drugs was better for the baby. And we thought we would have a big baby. When I said I didn't want drugs, my doctor supported me. We approached it as though it was a first birth, not a second, even though I knew all about being a mother and bringing a new baby home."

Not working, Liz was able to take good care of herself. She swam regularly and ate well. Her doctor kept tabs on Liz's fibroid, checking it at the beginning and end of the pregnancy. "We checked it three weeks before delivery," Liz recalled. "The doctor wanted to size the baby so we could see how big he was. The fibroid hadn't grown this time. It was still the size of an orange."

As her due date got closer, Liz knew this pregnancy was different. For one thing, the baby's head was down, and she had pressure on her bladder. She also experienced Braxton

Hicks contractions near her due date. Her labor started slowly. "I was casual about it," noted Liz.

All day Saturday, she was in mild labor. During a walk, her mother, who had come for the birth, noticed Liz pausing as a contraction passed. Then at 11 A.M. on Sunday morning, her water broke. "The mucus plug came out, and it was bloody," said Liz. "I couldn't tell if I was bleeding again or it was just a bloody plug." Her doctor told her to come to the hospital and determined that the mucus plug was bloody. He also found that Liz was four centimeters dilated.

"I would rather get to the hospital later," said Liz, who wanted to labor at home. "With VBACs, there are more hospital procedures that you have to pay attention to, and they watch the clock more. With a large baby, I didn't want a clock." At the hospital, Liz walked around for a few hours, trying to get her labor going. When that didn't work, the doctor suggested that he break Liz's water. "I didn't want him to, but he said, 'Let me do this.' If my labor took long, he might have to use other interventions. I trusted him," said Liz, who was pleasantly surprised to be in active labor 15 minutes after he broke her water. The downside was she also had to have an IV; it was a hospital requirement for anyone who had had her water broken.

Liz's labor took off after that. "The contractions were very intense. I could never get comfortable," she said. The nurses wanted to keep Liz attached to a fetal monitor. Liz wanted to move around. "I told the nurse that I had to keep moving. I said that I knew when I was having each contraction, so why did I have to be monitored in between?" Because Liz was insistent and able to articulate her concerns, she was able to strike a deal with the nurse: to be monitored for 10 minutes every hour.

"Before, I had been watching TV and chatting, but now I was concentrating on getting through each contraction," said

Liz. "I was in another world. Dan would crack a joke and I wasn't laughing. I thought, 'I can't do this anymore.' To me, the best part of Bradley were the signposts. When you couldn't stand the contractions any more, you were almost there."

At one point, another doctor came in, and Liz sent him packing. "I didn't want to meet someone new at this point." Liz's doctor popped in and out. Said Liz, "The life of an obstetrician is delivering babies, but they don't sit through the whole thing with you."

Liz got tired, lay down, and rested for 20 minutes. "All of a sudden, I had to go to the bathroom," she said. "I had an incredible urge to push. They got the doctor, he checked and said, 'Yes, let's go.' " Lest she get too excited, the doctor cautioned Liz that she might be pushing for a while.

"Pushing was great," she said. "Stirrups were comfortable for me, and I used them. I went for it as though I was running a race. I had control, and I liked that. I pushed for a little over an hour, but it felt like thirty minutes. I was almost there. I was doing great."

Then, because Liz was having a VBAC, she had to be moved from the birthing room to a delivery room—another hospital policy. (The fear is that stitches from the previous C-section would rupture.) "It was disruptive to have to move," said Liz. "I ended up in a different bed. It was stupid."

Once in the delivery room, Liz proceeded to push. Dan took out the video camera and began filming. "Everyone was cheering, the nurses and [the] doctor," recalled Liz. "Dan didn't need to be the support person anymore. He could videotape. I really went for it. They had a mirror, and I saw his head come out. I closed my eyes and pushed really hard, and all of a sudden I looked up, and there he was. It was great. I felt completely high and as happy as could be. It was amazing to me because I could hold him in my arms, nurse him. Within a little while, the IV was out, and I was walking to the bathroom. Dan couldn't believe it. With the C-section, I hadn't been out of bed for a while and needed recovery time. This was different."

For Liz, there was no comparison between the days following surgery and the days after her VBAC. "A VBAC is so much easier in terms of your health," said Liz. "But you have to be committed. You can't be halfway through and give up. You have to believe that it's okay to feel pain, it's part of the process. If you are not a person who can deal with pain, then go for something else. You have to figure out how to get through it.

"Giving birth is a very individual thing. It was a peak experience for me. The people at the hospital, the nurses and doctors, were so amazed. Why? Because I was so matter-of-fact. I did everything the way I wanted, and I did it without bullying them. I felt so good the next day."

✿ 18

Ivy's Story

Making the Second Time Better

Ivy Ratafia is under five feet tall. During her first birth, she fit into her doctor's under-five-foot-need-a-section rule. And she watched as the interventions started and the labor was taken out of her control. Ivy was determined that it wouldn't happen the second time.

Ivy Ratafia's first pregnancy got off to a medical start. She didn't conceive right away and sought the help of infertility specialists. By the time she conceived via in vitro fertilization (IVF), she was well educated about pregnancy. "I had been reading about pregnancy for those four years, waiting to get pregnant," said Ivy, who lived with her husband, Scott, in Massachusetts. "Then I read about infertility. Once I was pregnant, I read even more about pregnancy. That's what I did. I went to the library several times a week."

When she became pregnant, Ivy—a storyteller and actress in children's theater—left her job as a projectionist in a museum theater. Ivy had suffered from asthma for most of her life, so she'd been to a lot of doctors' offices. On top of that, there was her best friend's experience with open heart surgery. "I sat with my best friend through operations and recovery," said Ivy. "I had watched her and learned how to

155

deal with the medical profession—what one can accept and doesn't have to accept."

From the beginning of her pregnancy, Ivy wasn't thrilled with her prenatal care. She recalled one of her early doctor's visits. "When I went in for an appointment, I asked one of the [five] doctors [in the practice] about avoiding an episiotomy," said Ivy. "He told me that I had a four-in-ten chance, even a fifty percent chance, of having a C-section. I could try to labor for as long as I wanted, but he predicted that I'd be asking for a C-section."

Ivy believes that the doctor's opinion was based on her IVF conception. "They knew how much trouble I had conceiving. When the baby was two weeks late, they worried and didn't want anything to go wrong. They were fearful that this was our only chance. When the baby was late, they got nervous."

The doctors scheduled Ivy to be induced on a Thursday. They planned to use a gel to soften her cervix. Once labor started, they'd break her water. "We went to the hospital, and there were three emergency C-sections going on," recalled Ivy. "There was no room for us, and we were sent home. My contractions started that afternoon. We came back that evening and they did a nonstress test."

Ivy was pleased that labor was beginning on its own. "Things were starting to happen, and I was doing it myself." Ivy spent the next two days in mild labor; she lost her mucus plug and didn't sleep much. "I really thought I'd be able to labor," she said. "I thought, 'No intervention.' When I came back that evening, I thought we'd be able to leave, have dinner, and come back. But they wanted to keep me there all night. This is where the stupidity started. They wanted me to sleep, and they gave me morphine. I don't do well with drugs. I don't even take Tylenol. My body didn't take to it. I was suppose to sleep. Instead, it freaked me out. It was scary. It didn't make me sleepy. I couldn't walk to the bathroom myself. That's when I discovered how wobbly and shaky I was. I no longer had control over my body."

The woman in the other bed in Ivy's room had a friend with her. "They were talking softly, trying not to bother me," said Ivy. "But I was disturbed about them being there. They were making noise. The drug was doing things to my mind and body."

At 4 A.M., Ivy threw up her dinner. "I told the nurse that it was because of the drug," said Ivy. "But she said that the drug had worn off. I believe to this day that I was right."

Ivy was put into a birthing room, and they started the IV before her mother and husband were there. "I knew they would have trouble putting the IV in," said Ivy. Once she was on the IV, the doctor broke her water, but "Nothing happened. Then they gave me Pitocin. Because of the Pitocin, the contractions were painful. Because of the contractions, they had to monitor the baby, who seemed to be fine. I think the baby could have hung on for a few more days. I was determined to have natural childbirth, but under these circumstances, this wasn't natural."

A doctor came in, the one out of the five doctors in the practice whom Ivy didn't like. "I told him that I thought I was having back labor. He said, 'You've never been in labor before, so you don't know.' I wished I had said, 'You've never been in labor either. How do you know?' I was in pain. I was having back labor."

Because of the back labor, Scott "pounded" Ivy on the back. "He was my labor coach," she said, "hitting me on the back as hard as he could until I was black and blue." Finally, Ivy broke down and got epidural anesthesia.

"I didn't want the epidural," she continued. "I was in tears and exhausted. The epidural let me calm down and sleep, but it also slowed down my labor and then stopped everything. The contractions got farther apart. My body stopped at eight or nine centimeters. The baby hadn't engaged yet and was facing the other way. I was so drugged that I couldn't stand. Now there was no way gravity could help. The doctor had me lying in the bed anyway. That's why I finally gave in. I couldn't do anything to relieve the pain. I still get upset thinking about it."

The doctor decided that if labor didn't progress during the next hour, they'd do a C-section. Nothing happened. The contractions were seven minutes apart. The baby was still floating. "As far as he was concerned, he was right," said Ivy. "I was too small to have a baby. He didn't believe the baby was facing the wrong way.

"I was complaining about having a C-section, which was why the doctor gave me another hour," said Ivy. "My mom had been my birthing coach. She'd been with me all day. But my mom couldn't stand watching me. She thought it was best to get it all over with. I had been the one who had done all the reading. My husband and mother talked me into it. I think they respected my wishes, but they couldn't stand watching what I was going through. Everything caved in. I didn't have the fight left in me. It had been too long and too much. I was in tears, giving in to the operation."

Ivy was prepped for the operation. The anesthesia was made stronger, and she was shaved. Ivy and Scott had brought a CD player, and they put on Ivy's favorite song, "Zombie Jamboree" by Rockapella. The music, which was acapella, had lively lyrics about being "back to back" and "belly to belly." "It's a silly song and inappropriate," said Ivy. "I'd been dancing to it forever. I had been waiting to play it at the right time, a good time. So I hadn't played it yet."

When it was time for Ivy to be wheeled into the operating room, one of the nurses, who had been with her for hours, was going off duty. Instead, she decided to stay with Ivy so she could "see this thing through," said Ivy. "She had us singing the song ["Zombie Jamboree"] in the operating room. I calmed down every time I heard it. The music got me through," said Ivy. "The nurses got into it. They were singing with me. We were all singing. I listened to the song five times. This was the best part of the birth.

"I was conscious and scared to death," continued Ivy. "Boy, was I in bad shape. The nurse I liked stayed long enough for the baby to come out. It takes no time to get the baby out and a long time to get stitched up. They gave the baby to my husband, but then told him that I needed him more. He stayed and held my hand." Sky was born at 11:50 P.M., weighing 8 pounds 7 ounces.

After the operation, Ivy was shaking because of the drugs. "I just fell asleep and didn't really see my daughter until the next day," she said. "At one point, they woke me up and gave me Sky, and both of us were asleep. We didn't know what we were doing. We didn't nurse. There was nothing in me."

In the years that followed, Ivy learned to stop talking about Sky's birth. "It started to feel wrong," she said. "I didn't want to associate it with her. She was the good thing that came out of it. Some people have trouble disassociating the baby from the birth. I blamed it on the doctors. I knew that she [Sky] hadn't done anything wrong."

After she'd had time to reflect on the birth, Ivy began to realize what had gone wrong. "I was trusting. I had gone through infertility and had to fight for that to get what I wanted. The only reason I got pregnant was because I fought. I did a lot of work there. For the birth, I let them take over, even though I knew I shouldn't. It was something about going in late, being scared, and thinking maybe there was something wrong. I wasn't in the right frame of mind to disagree with anything. The whole thing was frustrating."

It took Ivy a long time to heal. She didn't think she could get pregnant again. "I hadn't gotten pregnant by myself the first time, and I thought it might take another four years. So we forgot about birth control." Three months later, she was pregnant.

Right away, Ivy made arrangements to see a midwife and changed to a health insurance plan that accepted her. Then she miscarried. Ironically, the same doctor who had delivered Sky was on call. "He wanted to give me a D & C, but I had been through enough," Ivy said. "I let myself miscarry. I was spotting and was bleeding. I drove out west and bled the whole way."

Ivy and her family moved to California. She continued to bleed lightly and finally went on the pill for three months, "the first intervention I'd let them do," she said.

Another three months went by and she was pregnant. By that time, Ivy and her family were staying with her parents in Newbury Park, between Santa Barbara and Los Angeles, waiting for Scott to sell his next project. "It was a difficult time financially," said Ivy. "We didn't have health insurance. No one will take on someone who is pregnant."

Ivy found a midwife in the area, 20 minutes away, who had her own birth center. But Ivy was upset by the birth record sent by the hospital. Written at the time of the operation, it included information about when Ivy had come to the hospital and then the C-section, but it didn't mention the hours in between. "It said that they had been planning to section me due to my size," said Ivy, who saw in the notes that Sky had been born facing backward, as she'd thought. But after Sky was born, at her first checkup, the doctor seemed to think that Ivy could have delivered vaginally—except for the way Sky was facing. "I was confused," said Ivy. "He seemed to change his mind, although at the time he didn't believe I had back labor."

Even without detailed records of her first labor, Ivy's midwife was all for her having a VBAC and wanted to know whether she wanted to have a home birth or to come to the birth center. "The birth center was better," said Ivy. "We were living at my parents' house, and it would have been difficult having a home birth there. Also, there was the fact that I was nervous." Even if she had had her own home, Ivy would have chosen the birth center because it was closer to the hospital if something went wrong.

Ivy heard great reports from other people about the midwife. As it turned out, the birth center was the only one in the area, and some people traveled there from as far as two hours away. "I had thought that California was so crunchy granola, yet she was the only midwife in the area," said Ivy. "If you went farther south or north, there were a lot. But not around here, which was why she was so busy."

The birth center was located in a Simi Valley strip mall, an outdoor mall with a restaurant on one side and offices on the other. The birth center had one big birthing room, with a tub and a bed, and other smaller rooms. Because the midwife's practice was so popular, if two patients ended up in labor at the same time, both had to come to the birthing center, even if one or both had been planning a home birth. That was the only way that the one midwife and her three assistants could take care of both women.

Ivy and Scott found out other peculiarities of the practice. For example, the midwife gave every woman Pitocin after delivery to prevent hemorrhage. "She did this as a matter of course," said Ivy. "I was going to talk to her about it, but I found out that she'd had a woman hemorrhage, and that's why she did it. I wasn't going to be able to talk her out of it. It was still too fresh in her mind."

Ivy did some research about Pitocin after birth. "I decided that the reason not to get Pitocin just seemed to be no intervention. I trusted her and decided to let her get away with it."

The midwife, a certified nurse-midwife, was more medically oriented than others. In California, certified nurse-midwives don't have hospital privileges, but this midwife had a license to practice at the birthing center and to do home births. She wasn't allowed to deliver breech babies, though.

161

(Ivy later found out that, by law in California, all breech deliveries must be done in hospitals.) Ivy grilled her about what would happen if something went wrong. "She would get her doctor to come with us to the hospital," said Ivy. "But she couldn't come with us. Her role would change from midwife to *doula* (labor-support person)."

Ivy didn't meet the doctor, although she would have liked to. "The midwife brushed me off on that one," said Ivy. "She didn't seem to think it was necessary.

"The midwife's biggest issue with me was that I had to relax. The way I relax is to ask questions over and over again. It looks like I'm uptight, but I'm actually relaxed."

Ivy decided not to have amniocentesis but agreed to ultrasound. (Because it was a VBAC, the midwife wanted to make sure that everything was all right.) "The technician had a headache and was having a bad day," said Ivy. "I couldn't see the screen, and no one said anything. I began to wonder if everything was all right. It turned out the baby was fine. I was very sick during the pregnancy, but I kept thinking that was a good thing. I hadn't been sick at all when I miscarried."

July 25, a Tuesday, was Ivy's due date. She had been having mild, not very painful contractions for the past week. There was a big annual convention that weekend that Ivy and Scott usually attended. "It would have been our tenth time at the convention," said Ivy. "We had been hoping the baby would come early, and we could go. But we couldn't." Instead, on Monday, friends who had attended the convention dropped by to visit.

That evening, they all went out to dinner. At the restaurant, Ivy's contractions got stronger. She went to the bathroom, and her mucus plug came out. "We spent the dinner timing contractions," she said. "They had become real. My husband had his pocket watch on a plate. I loved that."

Scott called the midwife when the contractions were six minutes apart. After the phone call, they were four minutes apart, lasting over a minute and getting more painful. It was about 10 P.M., and the midwife told them to come in at midnight. "I was nervous and thought we should go in sooner," said Ivy. "The midwife called back [when we got home] to say we could come in sooner. But it took us forever to get ready. Emotionally, I thought the baby wouldn't come like it hadn't last time."

At home, everyone was up. Sky woke up and wanted to come, and they took her with them. Ivy's mother and their friends also came along. They drove over in three cars. It turned out to be almost midnight by the time they got there.

"When the midwife saw everyone, she said, 'I'm just checking you. You're only one centimeter. I want to send you home.' I said, 'It's coming now.' I wanted to get in the tub. The midwife did another vaginal exam and, said, 'Let me see what I can do.' In one contraction, I went from one to three centimeters. I was soft and ready. And she said, 'Okay, you can stay.' "

Ivy still wanted to get in the tub, but the midwife didn't think she was ready. "She wanted me to walk around the waiting room," said Ivy. "Two minutes later, I threw up. This meant I was further along. She put me in the tub."

"Labor was harder than I thought it would be," said Ivy. "The first labor had been induced by Pitocin. I thought that was more painful than anything else I would go through. I'd gotten black and blue from it. I thought this labor wouldn't be as painful in the tub. I thought the water would make all the pain go away. It never got that horrible, but it was difficult. There were moments when I understood why people chose drugs. I didn't have the option at the birth center."

Sometimes there were a lot of people in the birthing room: Ivy's mother and husband, the midwife, and her assistant. The friends stayed with Sky in the waiting room. Every once in a while, Sky would come into the birthing room to tell her mother she loved her. Ivy took up a position lying on her side, facing a wall. She could hear people come in, but not see them. "I was alone with everyone there," she said.

The midwife checked Ivy a few times. About every 10 minutes, they listened to the baby with a stethoscope. Then Ivy would get back in the tub. At about 1:30, when Ivy was at six centimeters, the midwife wanted to break the water. "I said no, and she said, 'Okay.' It was up to me. It was too much intervention. I wanted to avoid breaking the water because of infection and the time factor. There was no reason for it. I had to say no to something. I had to have the control."

Again, at eight centimeters, the midwife wanted to break Ivy's water. This time, Ivy let her. She was feeling ready to push. "It felt different," said Ivy. "But the midwife's policy is that even once a woman has reached ten centimeters, she shouldn't push unless the baby is crowning. First, she told me to wait, and then she said I could bear down, and that made me happy."

Ivy and Scott barely had time to put a CD on the CD player. The midwife helped Ivy get out of the tub and brought her to the bed where she could put her in position to push—on her back, propped up, legs up. "I wasn't really pushing, but bearing down," said Ivy. "I really wanted to have the baby in the tub. But because I was a VBAC, the midwife was nervous."

It had been 15 minutes since the midwife broke her water. "I tore and then the head came out," said Ivy. "The midwife caught the baby. My mom and husband were right there. It had a huge effect on my mother to see her [grandchild] born. She kept saying, 'I saw her being born.' The whole thing was amazing. It happened so quickly. There was the work to get me out of the tub and onto the bed—the bed was high and I'm small. And then she was there." Ivy had arrived at the birthing center at 11:45 P.M., and Winter was born on August 1 at 2:10 A.M., weighing 7 pounds 8 ounces. "The midwife said that if I had let her break the water early, it would have been an even shorter labor," said Ivy, who held Winter immediately.

She was given a shot of Pitocin and delivered the placenta, which she saved and buried. "The idea of having something of her—the part of me that nourished her—nourishing something else seemed neat. It's planted under a tree."

Sky came in to meet her sister. Then everyone else came in to meet Winter.

Ivy and Scott spent the night at the birth center, the baby sleeping in between them. They went home the next morning, arriving before Sky was up.

Looking back, Ivy realizes that the pain involved in each of her two births was different. "I don't think there's such a thing as a painless birth," said Ivy. "The second one wasn't a breeze, but it was still great. It was a good kind of hard."

❧ 19

BETH'S STORY

A VBAC THAT CHANGED HER LIFE

Beth Curry's childbirth experiences changed her life. If her first birth, a C-section in a hospital, hadn't been so bad, she might not have had such a good second birth: a VBAC at home. Nor would she have become the childbirth reformer that she is today, as head of New Jersey Friends of Midwives. "Women are created to reproduce," says Beth. "This is a gift, like life is a gift. I don't see giving birth as a burden. If you've gone through natural childbirth without intervention, then you understand that gift. But when you take a woman and don't allow her to give birth or convince her that she doesn't want to, then you are taking something away that God gave her."

When Beth Curry of Freehold, New Jersey, was 26 and pregnant for the first time, she felt wonderful. "I wasn't afraid at all. I felt like I was walking around with God inside me, and I'm not a religious person. I thought it was the most amazing thing to be growing a person." This "like I was in heaven" feeling was not a surprise to Beth. She had always had her own outlook on life. "I've always looked at scenery from my own perspective. The colors are there, but most people don't see them. Most women think of pregnancy as just going to the doctor. I didn't see the inconvenience of it. Being pregnant is extrahuman. Men can't do it."

To prepare for her first birth, Beth read one book, Grantly Dick-Read's *Childbirth Without Fear*. This 1944 classic was one of the first books to introduce the idea of natural childbirth and the nonmedicalization of birth. The book gave Beth confidence. Because she wanted natural childbirth, Beth's sisters thought she was "living in a dream world. My labor plan was to find a female obstetrician. I assumed that I could tell her how eager I was to experience childbirth. As a woman, she'd understand what I meant. I went through pregnancy in ignorance. The doctor said, 'We'll see, we'll see' when I mentioned natural childbirth. She never said anything about anything. I thought, 'okay, if all goes well, she'll leave me alone.' "

In Lamaze class, the instructor noted that some class members might end up with a C-section; in fact, she predicted that three out of the ten women present would deliver that way. "Now, wasn't that inspiration!" said Beth. "But it [a C-section] wasn't going to happen to me. I felt healthy. I was taking good care of myself."

Being overdue was common with Beth's sisters, so she wasn't surprised when she went past her due date. When she was one and a half weeks late, she went to the doctor for a checkup. "The first thing she did was run her finger between the inside of the uterus and the back to loosen it. She did this without puncturing the sac. But she was very aggressive and she did it without asking me. I was naive and didn't ask questions." The exam hurt, and Beth felt uncomfortable when she left the office. (Six years later, when she did more reading about childbirth, Beth realized that her doctor had stripped her membranes. This procedure is done sometimes to get labor started when a baby is overdue.)

Early the next morning, Beth went into labor. At dawn, she called the doctor and was told to come to the hospital. Her husband Kent drove her there. From the time she arrived at the hospital, Beth was confused about the way she was treated. "I was either treated like an emergency or ignored. I handled the contractions all right. But sitting in a wheelchair felt worse."

When Beth was taken upstairs, the contractions picked up. She leaned over, the better to handle them. A nurse, watching Beth, suggested she do some "he-hes." "I didn't know what she was talking about. In Lamaze, you do that [the he-he breathing] at the end [of labor]. I wasn't good at breathing. I started hyperventilating. I started to faint. Now I was an emergency."

In seconds, Beth was hooked up to machines. 'What's in it?' I asked about the IV, while explaining that I didn't want any drugs. The nurse said, 'Don't worry, dear, it's just glucose water.' Twenty minutes later, I was screaming for painkillers. I thought I was going to die. It was the worst. The contractions were hell." Later, when Beth saw her hospital record, she found out that the doctor had put Pitocin in the IV (which was why her contractions were so painful).

Next, she was given epidural anesthesia. "I had felt fine when labor started. But now, for five hours, I lay there doing nothing." The doctor came in to do an exam and found that the baby's head was moulding (changing shape so it would fit through the pelvis) and there was caput (accumulation of fluid under the baby's scalp). (While neither moulding or caput is dangerous, it is sometimes an indication that the baby's head isn't going to fit through the pelvis.)

"Pitocin didn't make me dilate any faster," she said. "They wanted to go ahead and do the C-section." It was four in the afternoon and she'd been on the epidural for seven hours.

"They wheeled me down," said Beth. "I was nervous. You feel like a slab of meat. My arms and legs were shaking from nerves and the epidural. They had to tie my arms and legs down. I was glad because they were flying all around."

Kent wasn't in the operating room yet, and Beth was getting panicky. "I was learning that they don't always give you a straight answer. I was not going to go through this without my husband. Finally he came, and I felt better. There was nothing that had prepared me for this. It was the scariest moment of my life. Right before they began the surgery, I held my breath and jumped. I still had the feeling—my instincts were right—that I didn't need the surgery."

They increased the medication and Beth lost focus. "I felt sick and nauseated. I couldn't hear or see very much. I was hanging onto my life. I felt out of control."

Beth didn't feel them cut her open. But she could feel the tugging. Jonathan was born at 4:33 A.M. on April 21. "I don't remember hearing him cry. But I did hear the nurse say, 'You have a son.' "

The nurse's exclamation filled Beth "with joy. I'll never forget it. I tell him every year on his birthday how the nurse said this. That was the only good thing. It lasted a few seconds. They brought him over to me. My arms were tied down. I felt like I was ready to lose consciousness. All I could see was his mouth and nose. He was trying to nurse, and I couldn't do anything." Beth and Kent had agreed beforehand that if Beth couldn't take care of the baby or if anything happened to her, Kent would stay with the baby.

The anesthesia wore off, and Beth was in a lot of pain. She asked one of the nurses if she could have a painkiller and was told no. "I prayed that they would not bring me the baby. I was struggling so hard for myself. There was nothing I could do for him. I couldn't move. I spent about twenty minutes alone, afraid I would die." Finally a nurse came in and agreed to get the doctor; Beth was given some codeine.

A few years later, at an International Cesarean Awareness Network (ICAN) meeting, Beth remembered waking up in the hospital the morning after giving birth. "I was alone in the room. I looked out the window, and there was a pretty view. But I greeted the day all by myself. I felt so lonely, so horribly empty. I had never felt like this in my life. It was the first day of being a mother, and I felt so sad. That was my welcome to motherhood."

Later that morning, the nurses had the babies coming out of the nursery on a schedule. At about 10 A.M., they brought the babies to the mothers. "They brought a baby in. I sat up all excited to see my baby. And it wasn't my baby, it was my neighbor's. 'What kind of a mother am I?' I thought. I didn't know my own baby. I lost confidence. When childbirth is taken from you, it desensitizes you about trusting your own instincts and feeling confident about being a mother."

Her hospital experience, and the birth itself, affected her long after she got home. "I felt angry, and I was a monster to live with. I didn't know what I was angry about. I didn't even think I was angry about the C-section. People said I was so lucky to have a beautiful baby. How can you complain about having surgery if the result is a healthy, beautiful baby?"

After years of being angry and not knowing why, Beth started going to ICAN meetings. "I wanted another pregnancy. That's why I started going to the meetings. I'd always wanted a lot of children, one baby after another. But I didn't want to go through that experience again. When Jonathan was five, I heard little voices. 'But, mommy, I'm out here.' It took five years to hear these voices." At ICAN meetings, other women asked her questions about her birth, and she started to talk. She got angry and cried a lot.

Beth began to realize that it wasn't fair to her son to have such negative feelings about his birth. "It was my son's event, and it was a special event for me. I became more tactful about it. I had to adjust. I felt so injured and like such a victim. I've since learned to see the purpose in it. That it's not just negative. If I just talked about how negative it was, it wasn't fair to my son. It's not a nice thing for him, having a bad memory of his birth."

Beth convinced her husband to have another child. At first, he was against it and thought Beth was already too unhappy to cope with another child. "I needed to do it," she said. "He thought I was crazy because I was already so unhappy. But my plans and goals weren't reached yet. I wanted another baby. He finally gave in."

Beth got her medical records from the hospital. She interviewed doctors and visited hospitals. She tried to find midwives affiliated with hospitals. But at one hospital, for example, they said Beth wouldn't be able to use the birthing room because she'd had a C-section. "I needed all the advantages I could get. They wouldn't let me have the things I wanted." Beth found a hospital she liked but couldn't find a midwife there.

She began to feel as though "birth [in a hospital] was a political and financial issue. I didn't want any part of it. A birthing woman in a hospital is treated not as a person, but as an opportunity for a resident. It infuriated me. It was great; my anger took direction. Instead of being angry at my husband for not protecting me, and my son for not being the birth I wanted, I was angry at my hospital."

Beth read every book about childbirth she could find—and continued to dislike every hospital she visited. Meanwhile, when she was 34, she became pregnant again.

Someone lent Beth a book about the Bradley method, and she read it in one night. The next day, she knew what she wanted. "I had to have a home birth," she said. "That was the only way I could have the birth I needed. That was the way I'd be able to stay away from danger."

Through the grapevine, Beth found a midwife who did home births in her area. Getting this midwife to take her case became extremely important. There weren't many other choices available to her if she was to have the birth experience she desired. "I was so nervous when I called her," said Beth. "I felt as though I was wearing a scarlet 'C' for C-section. You're labelled. You feel discriminated against." Beth left a message to have the midwife call her back and spent hours near the phone, waiting for the call. "When I told her I'd had a C-section, I held my breath. She took me on. Finally somebody accepted me."

During the first prenatal visits, Beth didn't think she clicked with the midwife. This worried her; she felt as though the quality of her experience would depend on their ability to get along. "Hers was the only midwife practice around," Beth explained. "I had to get along with her and the rest of the midwives in her practice. It felt like having to get along with the nurses [at the hospital]. I anguished about it."

Then Beth stopped worrying. The midwife's office was big and open, and there was little privacy when seeing the midwife. As is common in some midwives' offices, women are encouraged to take care of themselves. In this office, each patient filled out her own chart, keeping track of heart rate and using a urine stick to check levels of protein and glucose in the urine (too much of either can cause a problem in pregnancy). Beth liked the way the women were encouraged to take care of their own bodies, that the midwives trusted them. During one visit, the midwife complimented Beth on how well she was taking care of herself. Finally, Beth was being praised for something she cared about. Another time, the midwife chastised Beth for saying negative things about Jonathan's birth in front of him. "She pointed it out to me. I'm glad she did."

For this birth, Beth took Bradley classes. "I really listened this time. They taught us how to negotiate [with the medical establishment]. It was good for me as a person. I learned how to ask for what was important to me."

The pregnancy went well, with no complications. But still the midwife wanted Beth to have a backup doctor because it was her first home birth. Again, it took Beth a long time to find a doctor she liked. Her task was made more difficult because she couldn't tell the doctor that she was really planning a home birth. Finally, she found a female doctor with hospital rights who seemed satisfactory. During one prenatal checkup there, Beth asked the doctor to use a stethoscope, not a Doppler (a form of ultrasound), to listen to the baby's heart. "She knew I was different. I'd been doing my own tests [at the midwife's]. She knew what I was doing." (Beth didn't even show up for her last prenatal visit. Two days after the birth, she called the doctor to say she was sorry she'd missed the last appointment, and she'd already had the baby. The doctor sent flowers, and Beth made sure she got paid for what she did. As it turned out, Beth was grateful; this doctor knew that she was planning a home birth and simply let her do it.)

Beth was anxious to feel labor again, but scared. She went past the due date but wasn't concerned. She went to a picnic with other families who had had home births and got a lot of advice from other mothers. At about the same time, Beth had a dream in which she and a girlfriend were being kidnapped. Each time the kidnappers cut her friend, Beth felt it. She had another dream in which little people were chasing her with knifes and cutting her legs.

She told her midwife about these dreams, and they joked about them. This made Beth feel better. "My midwife said, 'Birth is scary.' She also told me they don't do C-sections."

In the early hours of the next morning, Beth's labor began. She realized that she'd had to get those dream images "out of my thoughts" before labor started.

Jonathan, a first-grader, had been around a lot of other home-birth families. "He didn't want to see the baby born," said Beth, "but wanted to see her dressed. He wanted a sister."

That morning, Beth told Jonathan that the baby might be born that day. He could either stay home or go to school. Jonathan chose to stay home.

All morning, Beth's early labor didn't interfere with the family's activities, and, even though it was a weekday, it felt like a typical Saturday morning. Jonathan watched cartoons and colored. Beth gave Jonathan a bath. "We did regular weekend things," she said. "I did chores around the house and took a nap. We called friends and the midwives and told them I was in labor. We ate a big lunch." Early in the afternoon, they wanted to go out and do errands. They checked in with the midwives, who encouraged them to go about their normal activities. As Beth approached the car, she heard a pop, and her water broke. It was 12 hours after early labor had started.

Beth knew things were going to happen now. The contractions were getting more serious. She had Jonathan and Kent fill up the rented birthing tub with warm water. A half hour later, her labor really took off. "Now I was entering a different dimension," said Beth. "Suddenly I was only concentrating on the contractions." They called the midwives, who wanted to know the time between contractions. Beth didn't know but told them to come over. "I didn't want to be bothered thinking about anything. I realized in retrospect that last time, during heavy labor, I'd had to get my bag, drive to the hospital, register. It took energy from labor. This time I didn't have to think about anything. I put all my concentration into labor."

And that's what Beth did for the next eight hours. She put 100 percent effort into labor: going in and out of the tub, moving around the house, looking for comfortable places to labor. As it turned out, Beth had nothing to hold onto in the tub and didn't spend much time there. Jonathan and Kent were rushing around, getting things ready. "Jonathan didn't want to get near me. We weren't really helping each other at all." Beth took off her clothes because it was more comfortable without them on. She lay on her side, trying to relax and not work against the contractions.

Katie, Beth's friend and Bradley teacher, arrived. She was going to be the labor coach. "She walked into the house and the atmosphere changed—from nervous and apprehensive to relief. Here was someone who knew what was going on. Jonathan and Kent relaxed. Both of them were excited and worried.

"Jonathan went back to what he'd been doing. Katie said I looked great. That I was doing it. She started timing contractions, and they were two and a half minutes long, and not very far apart."

The midwives arrived but didn't have much to do with Beth at first. Katie and Kent took turns being with Beth. When Kent was there, Beth felt a little tense. "I knew the difference between Kent and Katie," she said. "I think a laboring mother needs a mothering figure—just like a baby can only fall asleep with its mother. A laboring woman knows that a woman, who is also a mother, makes her feel secure. It's a good idea to have a female labor coach. A woman can sense someone who's been through this. If it's a man, it's not the same thing. I'm glad I had Katie. It's a personality thing. I had enough people involved that I had what I needed when I needed it."

When the midwives examined Beth and told her she was at seven centimeters, she was thrilled. Someone commented on her "seven-centimeter smile," noted Beth. "I'd gotten past the five I'd gotten stuck at last time." Lying on her back during internal exams was uncomfortable for Beth. And it made her remember her previous birth, lying on her back in the hospital. "How do women do it? Going through labor, I felt close to all other women in time. It was corny, but I could feel empathy toward all those laboring on their back. I felt a connectedness to other women. Everything I experienced I know others have experienced."

Soon, Beth was dilated to 10 centimeters. "I knew that I'd be okay once I reached ten. I wasn't going to the hospital. I got really happy."

Beth began to feel a little urge within each contraction. She described it as a "resistance deep inside, not even the whole uterus. Within each contraction, that one resistance got a little bigger. It started as one centimeter, then five, then ten, until it was the whole uterus resisting, pushing against something. I wasn't pushing. The uterus was. You don't have to push, your uterus will do it."

The midwife checked to see if Beth could push without anything obstructing the baby's path. Up until then, Beth had been walking around the house, leaning over the end of the bed, the tub, the toilet. Several times she had climbed into bed. "I just wanted to get away from it," she said. "But that wouldn't work."

Pushing made Beth feel as though she was experiencing back labor. She felt the baby move down and the pain against her tailbone was excruciating. "I was thinking, 'I don't care if this baby breaks my back.' It hurt, but it didn't bother me. I felt heroic. Like everything was okay even if I broke a bone. It was still better than [being in] a hospital. I wasn't afraid of it. For that reason, I didn't hold back. I let it do anything to me. I had faith that everything would be all right."

Then the midwife could see the baby descending. "It was so wonderful to hear her say that, confirming what I was feeling," said Beth. "The baby was passing the tailbone. The midwives were so calm. It was supposed to happen this way." The baby got past that point, and the midwife could see 25 percent of the baby's head. She also said that in the old days, when she'd been an obstetrics nurse, the staff would call in the doctor when 25 percent of the baby's head was showing. "I loved hearing these stories," Beth said.

But the baby didn't come right out. "I was walking around, sitting on the toilet, feeling miserable. The midwife came in and asked, 'Well, what are you going to do next?' I said, 'I just need to feel comfortable.' She told me I wasn't going to get comfortable until I birthed the baby."

Beth asked her what she should do. The midwife suggested they go back into the bedroom. They suggested positions, and Beth tried them out. Then, the other midwife moved the furniture around and laid down towels on the floor. The baby's head was almost crowning. "I could feel the baby's head," Beth said. "They told me to touch it. I didn't want to see it in a mirror because when I walked I could feel it with my body. It was the most womanly feeling to have the baby's head almost out of my body. There's nothing that can match that feeling. I walked across the room with the head coming out of my body. The midwife was behind me. She put her hands under my arms and told me to hold onto her.

"On the next contraction, they told me to take a breath for myself and the baby and let it push. So I did. I felt very calm. I wasn't worried about the contraction getting too big. I took a breath for me and one for the baby." Beth squatted down, and felt a burning sensation as the perineum (the area between the anus and vaginal opening) was stressed. Beth didn't want to stop pushing, but the burning sensation made her want to.

On the next contraction, Beth used the same breathing technique. "The other midwife was on the floor in front of me. They were amazed that I knew when to stop pushing. It wasn't a lot of effort. I let the baby push. The head and shoulders came out. It was really quiet. No one said anything. On the next contraction, the rest of the baby slithered out like a fish, all wet. It was still quiet. The midwife caught her and let her to the floor. She lay on the floor face down."

Beth thought it was a boy. The midwife asked Beth if she wanted to hold her. "I got on my knees and looked at her. I turned her over. No one was doing anything. A hush. Jonathan had been watching from the corner of the room. At that point, he jumped up. He said he didn't want to see and ran out of the room. I was a little concerned about him, but not much. I turned her over. She was the most beautiful thing. A girl. It's a girl. We were so happy. We had all wanted a girl. She looked right at me. She looked at Kent. She looked at everyone around the room. No one said anything. Everyone looked at her, and she at us. Jonathan came back in, smiling. I picked her up and held her. We spent minutes looking at her. The first thing I noticed was that she looked like Jonathan."

" 'Meet your sister,' I said to Jonathan. That was the biggest moment of my life, to have my two children. I recognized Jonathan in her face right away. I was so glad Jonathan wanted to be there. I couldn't give him that kind of birth, but I could give him his sister's birth. I was glad that he'd had that. I think it was worth it."

Emily's birth helped Beth with Jonathan. "I didn't want him away [from us]. I told him if he wanted to sleep with us, he could. That was the first thing. Now that he was six, he said he was fine on his own. We didn't have expectations of him anymore. When he had nightmares, he would wake us up. After Emily was born, I would sit and rock him. We'd talk about the nightmares. I became more concerned about him. When he was younger, I wasn't very sympathetic to him because I felt like other people didn't care about my feelings. It got pushed off on him."

A half hour after Emily was born, Beth took a shower. "It felt wonderful. I enjoyed the steam and the hot water." The midwife was standing outside the shower with a towel for Beth. "She dried me," she said. "I felt like a queen. I felt royal. I don't know why. Her background was nursing. That was the kind of thing you do for a woman who has just given birth. It reminded me of stories in the Bible. The midwife was there to serve the birthing woman. They honor the birthing woman. And I felt honored."

After Emily's birth, Beth also felt as though her husband treated her differently, too. "He honored me also," she said. "He found a new kind of respect for me, with what I'd done." For a week, Kent took care of Beth, doing the cooking and cleaning, so she could rest and nurse the baby. "I learned to respect him for doing this," said Beth. "We learned a great respect for each other. When we have hard times, we think about when Emily was born. We still have that respect for each other from that time."

Beth called her mother. "It was just like any other phone call. I told my mom I was doing great. That I was lying here with my new daughter. She screamed." Beth told her mother not to come immediately. Beth and Kent wanted to be alone with their children. "I didn't want anyone interfering with our family," she said. "We lay around in bed. Kent took care of us. Jonathan helped. We put up the heat so the baby wouldn't get cold. It was just our family. The midwives came to visit. They were courteous of the way we did things in our home."

The midwives told Beth they were especially pleased with her birth. "They had seen me as insecure and angry," said Beth. "I had a lot of things to work out. They saw my husband as not being supportive. I've learned about him. I don't push him. I go my way and he goes his. He is not supportive at the beginning. He takes a while to warm up."

When Beth's mother arrived, she couldn't stop telling Beth how to do things, but she also observed a lot. When one of Beth's sisters asked whether postpartum depression had hit yet, Beth's mother admitted there was no evidence of postpartum depression, and that maybe it had to do with her having the baby at home. Beth could tell her mother was beginning to think there might be something to this "home-birth thing."

Beth's childbirth experiences have influenced the rest of her life. She has even realized the importance of Jonathan's birth. "Having both kinds of births gave me experience," said

Beth. "Some women haven't had a C-section. I experienced it. I know what they've gone through. The C-section was a valuable experience personally and professionally. I don't regret it, although I don't advise other people to go that route. I work to help women avoid these experiences. I don't want them to suffer the way I did. It's unnecessary."

Because of her VBAC, Beth's relationship with her husband and her son changed, as did her feelings about herself. In her file at the hospital, someone in admissions had noted on the form that Beth was "meek." "That's how I was," said Beth. "But not anymore."

PART FIVE

How You Can Have a Joyful Childbirth

20

PUTTING THE PIECES IN PLACE FOR A POSITIVE EXPERIENCE

If there is anything that's clear from these birth stories, it is that childbirth is an unpredictable experience. There are few things in life that are so unknown.

Many factors play a role in how labor and delivery will go: the size of the baby, the size of your pelvis, and the position of the baby. It is also known that the release of the hormone oxytocin is important in helping labor begin. But there is no way to know when labor will start (or, in some cases, whether it will begin at all).

Some women say, "But I did everything I could to prepare for childbirth." They ate well, exercised, and had regular prenatal checkups—and then were surprised when labor didn't go as planned. Of course, taking good care of yourself is an important, and necessary, part of pregnancy. But, unfortunately, this will not ensure that your childbirth experience will also go according to plan.

Most likely, you will not be able to anticipate your reaction to every aspect of labor, nor will you be able to completely prepare for it. (This may be difficult for some women who are used to controlling everything in their lives.) But you can prepare yourself and make careful choices about how you want to give birth, with whom, and where.

What makes a satisfying childbirth experience? In her book *Obstetric Myths Versus Research Realities*, Henci Goer cited studies from 1981 that point to *mastery*—having a sense of control during childbirth—as the main reason for women's satisfaction during childbirth. A 1994 Australian study by Stephanie Brown and Judith Lumley expanded on this. Looking at satisfaction in labor and birth, these researchers found that being informed, participating in decision making, and developing relationships with caregivers influenced women's satisfaction.

"Women who have had positive birth experiences usually feel as though they had some control over their births," said Linda Maldanado, a labor-support professional in Riverdale, New York. "If they needed a drug, they knew what they needed and got it, and they used machines, like the fetal monitor, to their advantage." Let's look at how you can do this.

KNOW YOURSELF

Although natural childbirth might be the ideal for many, it is not everyone's first choice, nor is it always a reality for those for whom it *is* the first choice. Maybe, in the future, when women know more about obstetrics and their own bodies, more will choose natural childbirth. However, with today's vast array of options, each woman must make decisions about giving birth.

In preparing for *your* childbirth experience, consider who you are. Take into account your own personality and preferences. If you really think about it, you will discover views and

184

feelings about yourself that will indicate the kind of childbirth experience with which you will be most comfortable. You have come into pregnancy and childbirth with these feelings. Think about what you like and don't like. Reflect on past medical experiences: How did you react? Have you had good experiences with doctors and hospitals? Have you dealt with doctors you trust? Does your family treat you with dignity when you are ill or like a baby? Which kind of treatment are you used to? Which do you like?

Anthropologist Robbie Davis-Floyd, in her book *Birth as an American Rite of Passage*, explained that there are two main ways of thinking about childbirth, two ways that "represent opposite ends" of the pregnancy and childbirth spectrum. Wrote Davis-Floyd, "The holistic model is fundamentally different from the technocratic model—to fully believe one is to fully disbelieve the other." The basic idea of Davis-Floyd's paradigm goes like this:

Technocratic	*Holistic*
Using technology	Relying on experiential or emotional knowledge
Doctor	Midwife
Medical intervention necessary	Medical intervention unnecessary

Realize that as these birth stories indicate, there is fluctuation within the paradigm. For example, there are midwives working at hospitals, and doctors with low C-section rates. A painkiller can sometimes allow a woman to experience the moment of birth. To put it in Davis-Floyd's terms, the single factor that "most influences the conceptual outcome of a woman's birth" is the relationship between what happens to her during childbirth and the belief system she holds. You have to know what you think.

Define your belief system by analyzing what you think and by identifying your basic reactions and gut instincts—these will guide you toward the childbirth experience, including the caregiver and birth setting, that's best for you.

You are probably more comfortable giving birth in a hospital with a doctor as caregiver if:

- You feel that technology enables you to experience labor with less pain.
- You feel most comfortable in a hospital.
- You have a high regard for doctors.
- You're more comfortable in a setting where there is emergency medical assistance if you need it.
- You're worried about your ability to handle pain.

You are probably more comfortable giving birth in a non-hospital setting, a setting that is less conducive to interventions, with a midwife as a caregiver if:

- You feel as though using drugs will make you feel strange and contribute to the feeling that you are ill or immobile.
- You're concerned about the effects of drugs on your unborn child.
- You don't believe giving birth should be treated as an illness.
- You have a high regard for midwives.
- You feel most comfortable in a nonmedical environment where you feel in control and at ease.
- You would like someone beside your husband to be with you throughout the labor and delivery.
- You believe in your body's ability to give birth naturally.

Your reaction to these statements will begin to give you a clue about the kind of childbirth experience with which you'll be most comfortable.

DO RESEARCH

Be as informed as you can be about what childbirth is like. Many women read as many books as they can. They also ask new mothers about their childbirth experiences.

"I know a lot of women who want a wonderful birth experience but don't want to make the effort," said Heidi Rinehart, M.D., an obstetrician in Glendale, Arizona. And it does take some effort. When Beth Curry gave birth for the first time, she read one very encouraging book about childbirth and assumed that with a female obstetrician she'd have no problem experiencing the birth she wanted. Now she's the first one to say how wrong she was. She educated herself so completely before giving birth the second time that she became involved in childbirth reform.

FIND OUT ABOUT YOUR MOTHER'S LABOR

You'll notice in these stories that a woman's childbirth experience is often compared to her mother's or sister's. This is because it is generally believed that you are built in a similar way to your mother or sister and that your body might handle childbirth the same way. Your caregiver might ask you questions about childbirth experiences in your family as a possible indication of how your own will go.

My labor was long and slow and had several stops and starts. My mother always used the term "false labor" when referring to her early, slow contractions. One woman explained that, during an early prenatal exam, her midwife noted that she had an unusually narrow pelvis; it turned out that her mother had the same body structure. Annette Cantor's mother had given birth at home, so it seemed only natural to Annette to do the same. Unmedicated births and home births were also the fashion in Rosemary Moore's family, so even though she was having twins, she believed she could birth them naturally, or at least had the encouragement and support to try.

Ask your mother—or other women on your side of the family—about their childbirth experiences and the size of their babies. It can't hurt to find out how labor and delivery went for them, and it might just help you find out more about your own. Look at the other side of the gene pool, too. Was your husband a big baby? Even though she was not tall, Megan Howard knew big babies ran in her family. When Jed was born, he kept that family tradition going.

TAKE A GOOD CHILDBIRTH CLASS

The goal of taking childbirth classes is to find out more about the experience you're about to have. It is generally believed that women are less fearful about labor and delivery when they know what to expect. Classes usually inform couples about the different stages of labor and teach relaxation techniques, proper breathing, and exercises that prepare for childbirth. They also might teach about the kinds of painkillers and epidurals offered. A session or two might be devoted to what happens during a C-section. (Many women don't attend this session because they don't think they'll have a C-section. Some are sorry they didn't.)

The most common classes available to women in this country are Lamaze, Bradley, and the International Childbirth Education Association. ICEA's course is a combination of many kinds of childbirth education, and as part of its goal it stresses family-centered maternity care.

When the Lamaze method was first introduced in this country in the late 1950s, twilight sleep was in its heyday. (Twilight sleep was a technique for painless birth in which a woman received morphine and an amnesiac drug, which caused her to forget what was happening.) The Lamaze method came along and allowed women to be awake during the birth, which, after twilight sleep, was a big change. In the early years, Lamaze focused on breathing techniques and mental exercises designed to distract a woman from the pain of birth. As labor progressed and the contractions got more intense, so did the breathing patterns. Recently, Lamaze has been criticized because, in using this method, a laboring woman tries to control her own behavior but has little say in medical decisions made on her behalf.

One of the main tenets of the Bradley method is that women need to understand what's happening in their body during each stage of labor, the better to relax and go with the flow of labor. Bradley encourages normal breathing in labor and teaches systematic relaxation. Bradley also promotes the idea of the husband as labor coach. In many Bradley classes, there is an opportunity to discuss individual doctors and hospitals, and the instructor shares information about how you can expect to be treated at a particular hospital and what you can do about this treatment. "You have to be street-smart," said Doris Haire, director of the American Foundation for Maternal and Child Health in New York City, about childbirth education. "Many instructors teach to make the doctors happy. I tell people to go to a Bradley class. They are more honest about the risks."

Childbirth instruction varies greatly depending on where you take the class and with whom. It's a good idea to shop around to find out about childbirth educators in your area—specifically, what and how they teach. Many hospitals offer childbirth education classes, or you can contact a local childbirth education organization. (See the Resource list at the back of the book for information about childbirth educators.)

Are all the pieces in place? Next, you'll need to focus on choosing a birth place and a caregiver.

✿ 21

CHOOSING THE BIRTH PLACE

What do you do first when planning to give birth—
choose a birth place or a caregiver? Many women simply
stay with their current obstetrician/gynecologist. Others
start interviewing new physicians and midwives. But it is
the place where you give birth that dictates the kind of caregiver you're looking for. That's because caregivers at hospitals and birth centers follow that place's rules and guidelines about maternity procedures, such as requiring IVs and
electronic fetal monitoring. Many hospitals, too, will have
different C-section rates. If you choose a hospital with a low
rate, it stands to reason that your chances of having a
cesarean will be lower than at a hospital with a high rate.
Even if you are insured by an HMO and must choose from
a specific list of practitioners, you can find out about the
available birth places in order to assess the kind of childbirth
experience offered at each.

It is important to note that there are choices about where
to give birth—hospital, birth center, or your own home. Despite these options, most women deliver in hospitals. In fact
the U.S. Department of Health estimates that 99 percent of all

191

babies born in the United States are born in hospitals, and this had been the case since 1975.

It wasn't always this way in America. Before the mid-1800s, most women gave birth at home and were assisted by other women. In those days, it was believed that giving birth at home was safer because maternity wards were full of disease and infection. Then around 1850, there was a move toward the medicalization of birth. It was viewed as a status symbol to give birth in a hospital. The trend toward hospital births also resulted in the development of new technologies to assist labor, the creation of the specialty known as obstetrics, and the passing of power from midwives to professional men. It might also have resulted in the feeling many women have that birth is a medical condition, rather than an experience in which women have options and can have a rewarding experience.

Where you choose to give birth is a personal decision and has to do with where you feel most comfortable.

HOME BIRTHS

Although less than one percent of all women in America give birth at home, it is a viable choice for some. (In some other countries, such as the Netherlands, as many as 40 percent of all births take place at home.) Annette Cantor wanted to give birth at home because she wanted to be in her own environment. She knew there were rules at a hospital that must be observed, and she wanted to choreograph the birth her way. Beth Curry chose to have her second birth at home because she felt safer there. After having her first child in the hospital, she felt as though the only place where she'd really have control over her birth was at home.

As these women's stories reveal, a woman laboring at home can do whatever she wants—have a cup of tea, move in and out of a birthing tub, walk around outside, have any number of people there to help. If labor doesn't progress or the baby is in distress, the midwife advises the woman to go to a hospital, as in the case of Sarah Ryan.

According to Henci Goer, there have been no studies that show excess risk when women with a trained attendant taking the right precautions attempt a planned home birth. As Goer points out, this option "is a matter of individual choice. The real question about safety is not, 'Do you want a pleasant birth at home or a safe birth in the hospital?' It is 'Do you want to give birth at home and run the minuscule risk of an emergency that might (but not necessarily would) be handled better in the hospital, or do you want to give birth in the hospital and run the considerable risk of infection, the certainty of additional stress, and the near certainty of having unnecessary (and potentially risky) interventions?' "

BIRTH CENTERS

The U.S. Department of Health estimated that in 1993, 0.3 percent of all births occurred at freestanding birth centers. There are about 140 birth centers operating in this country (and about 105 more are being developed). They offer a homelike atmosphere in which to deliver. Most birth centers are either run or operated by certified nurse-midwives.

Birth centers are relatively new. The first one, the Maternity Center Association in New York City, was opened in 1975. According to the National Association of Childbearing Centers, birth center births are less expensive than hospital births. In 1993, the average birth-center charge was $3,268, while hospital charges averaged $5,436. The National Birth Center Study published in 1989 found that women at birth centers have a low cesarean rate of 4.4 percent, about one-half that of studies of low-risk, hospital births.

"A lot of traditional labor and delivery units in hospitals have rocking chairs and call themselves birth centers," said Susan Stapleton, president of the National Association of Childbearing Centers. "But birth centers are separate from hospitals. They are houses or offices designed to be homelike. Sometimes they look like bed-and-breakfasts. We do not provide epidurals, IVs, or C-sections, but do have the capacity to offer pain medication, even though we don't often need to offer it. We do other things, such as have a midwife continuously with a laboring woman, and let that woman do whatever her body tells her."

Although fewer births occur in birth centers nationally compared to hospitals, birth centers could play an important role in the future. "This setting remains of considerable interest as a safe and cost-effective alternative to hospital delivery for low-risk women," advised the Centers for Disease Control and Prevention Monthly Vital Statistics Report.

HOSPITALS

Today, the majority of women in America deliver in hospitals. Many feel safe there, knowing that all the medical technology they need is available. I know one mother, a pediatrician, who said that she'd spent so much time working in hospitals that she felt more comfortable giving birth there than in her living room. Similarly, Val Harper, who had so much knee surgery, knew what to expect in the operating room and what it felt like to recover from surgery.

Not all hospitals are alike. As these birth stories reveal, each hospital has its own policies regarding labor and delivery.

194

Some are more strict and require that IV and electronic fetal monitoring be used at all times. Some hospitals are affiliated with midwifery practices. Others don't allow midwives to practice there at all.

Remember, too, that the practitioner you choose and the birth place in which that practitioner delivers usually go hand in hand. That's because a site's procedures and policies dictate how a practitioner delivers there. If a doctor requires an IV and a fetal monitor, chances are the hospital where she delivers does, too. Similarly, a hospital in which midwives practice is more accustomed to unmedicated labors. Understand that, like doctors, hospitals can differ greatly in their approach to labor and delivery.

In finding out how maternity procedures are handled at your local hospital, you might get different answers from different people. A hospital public relations office might have glossy brochures that describe the hospital's maternity wing. Their answers to your questions might differ from an obstetrics, nurse or labor coach, for example, who has knowledge of what really goes on on the labor floor. Through childbirth instructors, labor coaches, and mothers who have given birth there, you should begin to get a sense of what giving birth in a particular hospital is like.

Here are some questions you can ask about the hospital you are considering. It is up to you to decide whether or not you're comfortable with their answers.

Is an IV given routinely?

Will I be shaved and required to have an enema?

Will I be hooked up to a fetal monitor for the entire labor?

Can I walk around and move freely during labor?

Do you have birthing rooms and delivery rooms? Is there a difference? Who gets which?

Can I eat and drink during labor?

How many people can I have in the room with me while I'm in labor?

Can my other children be present during the birth?

Are there reasons (such as a VBAC or other medical condition) why I might be moved from a birthing room to a delivery room in the middle of labor?

What is your C-section rate?

If a C-section is necessary, can my partner stay with me?

If I have a C-section, can the baby be in the recovery room with me?

What is your episiotomy rate?

Can the care that's given the baby after birth be done in the room where I am, or must the baby be taken away for routine procedures?

Can my baby remain with me immediately after the birth?

Is there rooming-in? Can my baby stay in the room with me at all times?

If there is no rooming-in, can my baby be brought to me at any time, or is the baby kept on a schedule?

Is there a lactation consultant on staff?

Mothers say that being treated with respect and dignity during labor and delivery contribute to their positive experience. To find out whether the hospital staff is courteous and respectful to laboring women, ask your caregiver for the names of other women who have delivered there. Ask them about their experiences, but be prepared for the fact that what you hear about is not always what you get.

I gave birth in a hospital that had a staff with a reputation for being helpful and courteous. But the hospital was extremely busy when I was there. After delivering, there was no room available for me, and a makeshift space was created for me in the nurse's lounge until I was able to have my own room.

The maternity floor was short-staffed during my stay, and I did not receive the wonderful treatment I'd heard about.

Tal Recanati believes that the Portland Hospital for Women and Children, where she delivered in London, provided a luxurious, calm atmosphere that helped her through her experience. She says it was a lovely place to have a baby. Rosemary Moore and Kari Garcia Fisher, who gave birth in hospitals in New York City, and Vicki Placha, who delivered in a Salt Lake City hospital, give a lot of credit to the staff and nurses for providing assistance and empathy.

NAVIGATING YOUR WAY THROUGH A HOSPITAL BIRTH

During one of my Bradley classes, the instructor asked each couple for the name of their doctor and the place where they planned to give birth. The instructor, who was intimate with the details of hospital policies and doctors' strengths and weaknesses, was able to warn each couple about what they might be up against. She knew which hospitals were inflexible about their policies regarding IV, Pitocin, or fetal monitoring, for example; she knew which doctors didn't let you squat or stand during the pushing phase. And she gave each couple tips on how to negotiate at each hospital—with whom and when and what was worth fighting for. She provided information about how other couples had fared and on dealing with the hospital staff. It's too bad that, in 1991 in the United States, 10 couples needed that kind of advice. But the bottom line is we did.

Ask friends or other women how they bargained with hospital staff, or if they had to. Liz Benson struck a deal with the nurses about how often, and how long, she had to be monitored. This gave her the opportunity to move around during labor.

For women who do not have a high-risk pregnancy, midwives and doctors offer this important piece of advice: Don't get to the hospital too early. During the early phase of labor, when labor is manageable, women are often more comfortable at home—where they can eat what they like and move around as they like. By not arriving at the hospital too early, women avoid being offered drugs or painkillers too early in labor.

From childbirth educators and other new mothers, find out whether your doctor or hospital staff is in the habit of honoring birth plans. Even if you've written down what you want (and had your doctor sign it ahead of time) and distributed it, the staff might be too busy to pay attention to your requests. In the middle of labor, you might be feeling vulnerable and not have the energy to argue about what you want.

WHAT TO KNOW ABOUT PAIN, PAINKILLERS, AND EPIDURAL ANESTHESIA

Drugs: The issue of whether or not to use drugs during labor is a big one for many women. Some know that they want a painkiller or epidural during labor. Others feel that they don't want anything. But, as many caregivers and childbirth educators state, you might not know what you really want until you're in labor.

Miriam Block wanted, and planned for, natural childbirth. But epidural anesthesia enabled her to get through a long labor and to experience (and enjoy) the actual moment when her daughter was born. If you had asked Miriam about her plans for delivery early on in her pregnancy, an epidural would have been one of the furthest things from her mind.

Because you can't be sure what labor will bring, it's a good idea to have an understanding of the kinds of painkillers and epidurals available and of how using these tools could affect your labor and your baby. Or, if you must make a decision to use drugs during labor, it's an informed choice.

Some women are able to avoid using drugs by having an idea about what the pain is and what it does for them during labor. "The pain and stress of normal labor have value," wrote Henci Goer in *Obstetric Myths Versus Research Realities*. She noted studies that showed that the stress hormones "produced in response to labor" help prepare the baby to breathe, use fuel for energy, and protect the baby against lack of oxygen during labor. "Pain guides the mother," wrote Goer. "Commonly, the positions and activities she chooses for comfort are also those that promote good labor progress or help shift the baby into the right position for birth. Remove the pain, and you kill that feedback mechanism, too."

Midwives and labor coaches often have nonpharmacologic methods of pain relief up their sleeves to suggest. Some of these are taking a warm shower or bath, massage, or walking or changing position. When my labor slowed down around seven centimeters, my midwife told me that I had several choices. She could break my water—which would probably make the labor pick up—or I could get into the position that was most uncomfortable and I'd been avoiding. It was a suggestion; it was up to me. Of course, I assumed the hated, on-my-side position. But it did what she said it would do. It got me into transition.

"The best way to avoid unnecessary drugs is to be prepared, have support, and make a good-faith effort to try nonpharmacologic means of pain relief," suggested Samantha McCormick of the International Cesarean Awareness Network in New York City.

What if you really feel you must have a painkiller or epidural? Just be aware of what you're getting yourself into.

Drugs are known to slow down labor. Often, epidural anesthesia interferes with a woman's ability to push the baby out herself. Any time you have a painkiller or epidural, you must be hooked up to an IV—which inhibits your ability to move around during labor. (Remember that moving around during labor is a great form of nondrug pain relief.) Once you start using any kind of intervention, it is much more likely that you will need to rely on another, and another. And, thus, the daisy chain of events has started. This is what happens when many women feel as though their labor is taken away from them. This is how they begin to feel that they lose control.

Not only could your labor be affected by drugs, but so, too, could your baby. Doris Haire, director of the American Foundation for Maternal and Child Health in New York City, has done extensive research on obstetric drugs. As she wrote in *The Encyclopedia of Childbearing,* "Seldom are pregnant women advised by their obstetricians that an unborn baby's central nervous system is rapidly forming throughout the latter months of pregnancy, the perinatal period, and the first two years of life, and that during that time, the central nervous system is susceptible to permanent damage from drugs prescribed for or administered to the pregnant women." As Haire noted, more research needs to be done on the long-term effect of these drugs.

Taking into account what we know about drugs—and their effect on labor and the baby—what do childbirth experts and practitioners advise? Use painkillers and epidurals if you really can't cope without one, but be aware of the possible consequences.

In her book *Your Baby, Your Way,* British childbirth educator Sheila Kitzinger also maintained that "drugs for pain relief have a definite place in childbirth—especially when there are deviations from the normal and a woman is in severe pain. There is no need for any woman to prove her womanhood by laboring without drugs when she is experiencing more pain than she is prepared to cope with."

PAINKILLERS

Notice how the women in these birth stories reacted to the painkillers they took. Susan Bjornson was given Demerol, a drug frequently given in labor to "take the edge off." She had been laboring without dilating for hours and believes that the drug allowed her to rest and relax. She was then able to resume labor. She said Demerol prevented her from having a C-section. But other women who are given Demerol report that it can make them confused or make them feel as though they are having one big contraction.

Miriam Block was given Nubain, a narcotic-like drug, when she was exhausted and in the middle of a long labor. Unlike Susan Bjornson's reaction to Demerol, Miriam's labor changed when she was on the drug. She lost touch with why she was in the hospital and having contractions. She couldn't labor properly because she was so busy coping with the effects of the drug.

Both Demerol and Nubain and other analgesic drugs (which relieve pain) can cause side effects such as nausea or vomiting, headache, or sweating. Sometimes women are given a second drug in conjunction with the first to reduce these side effects.

The problem with taking a painkiller is that you won't know how you'll react to it until after you've taken it. It's a good idea to have several thorough conversations with your caregiver about the painkillers she recommends. (See Chapter 22 for general questions to ask your caregiver.) When it comes to drugs, you'll want to find out which ones might be offered and when. Ask about drugs used for induction and when these would be given. Ask what effect the drug might have on labor and on the baby. You can also ask about dose: Is it possible to have a very small dose at a time? Do you have any choices about which drug you take? Are any nonpharmacological pain relief techniques recommended before you're given the drug?

EPIDURAL ANESTHESIA

There are different kinds of anesthetics. General anesthesia renders a person unconscious; it is used for emergency C-sections or when a doctor wants a woman to be unconscious during the birth. Regional anesthesia numbs an area of the body; in this case, the lower body.

Regional anesthesia can be administered in different forms, including epidural, caudal, pudendal, or spinal anesthesia. As you've seen in these stories, some women refer to regional anesthesia is general terms, often using the word *epidural* to mean any kind of regional anesthesia. Women who have C-sections and are awake for the births also receive a form of regional anesthesia. How do the various forms of regional anesthesia differ? A *pudendal block* numbs the woman's perineum and is usually given right before birth occurs. *Spinal* anesthesia (often used during C-sections) is injected into the fluid near the spinal cord and numbs the body from the chest down. *Caudal* anesthesia is injected below the bone in the small of the back and numbs less of the body than the spinal. *Epidural* anesthesia is injected into the middle or lower back and only numbs the most painful area. When epidural anesthesia is administered with great care, it is possible for some women to still have feeling in their legs, allowing them to push and participate in the actual birth.

Some women seem to have positive experiences with epidural anesthesia when they receive it at the right time and are still able to participate in the birth of their child. Both Vicki Placha and Miriam Block were able to participate in the pushing stage of labor because the anesthesia was given at the right time and in the right amount and then wore off at the right time. The change in Miriam's strength and her ability to labor is particularly noticeable because she was so out of control on Nubain. Her epidural allowed her to rest and then to participate in—and enjoy—the birth of her daughter.

It's a good idea to find out your caregiver's opinion about epidural anesthesia and what types are given. Some doctors use them routinely. Others don't. Find out how many of your caregiver's patients get epidurals. You can also ask when they are given; for example, a doctor might have a general rule about waiting to give an epidural until a woman has dilated to a certain point. Understanding your caregiver's use of this drug will help you during labor.

Epidural anesthesia is not for everyone. "If a woman is progressing well, all she needs is encouragement to go on," says Carol Bronte, a certified nurse-midwife in New York City. "Epidurals are for people who are fatigued and not progressing."

In 1987, Sheila Kitzinger noted in "Some Women's Experiences of Epidurals: A Descriptive Study" that when epidurals work well, women are satisfied with their childbirth experience. In *The Encyclopedia of Childbearing*, she wrote, "They reported tremendous relief from pain and a renewed sense of control. Many of these women have good relationships with their caregivers and were free of constraints either to have drugs or to manage without an epidural. All of the women who were entirely positive about their experience of birth with an epidural felt free from pressure to have the epidural."

WHY C-SECTIONS HAPPEN

About one fourth of all births in this country are cesarean sections. Before 1970, C-sections were used as a last resort, and the rate nationally was about 5.5 percent. Since the mid-1970s, the C-section rate has risen gradually, reaching 24.7 percent in 1988, which is one of the highest C-section rates in the world. Because of this "epidemic," the Centers for Disease Control and Prevention is urging reduction of the C-section rate to 15 percent by the year 2000 as one of its main health-promotion objectives.

It is common for some obstetricians to defend the high C-section rate by pointing to the decline in the U.S. perinatal mortality rates. But many healthcare experts believe that other factors are really responsible for this decline: better prenatal care and nutrition, better prenatal education, and advances in care for premature babies. "Many industrialized nations have lower perinatal and infant mortality rates than the United States, yet most have C-section rates less than half as high as ours," wrote Mary Gabay and Sidney M. Wolfe, M.D., in *Unnecessary Cesarean Sections*.

In some cases, such as placenta previa (a rare event that involves the placenta partially blocking the opening to the uterus), C-sections are the safest way to have a baby. According to this report, the four reasons for 86.3 percent of all cesareans in 1991 were not these rare conditions. The four main reasons were:

1. A previous C-section—It is often assumed that women who have had cesareans will automatically have another one.
2. Dystocia—This is the medical term for abnormal labor, for example when the baby's head seems to be too big to

fit through the mother's pelvis. It also refers to prolonged labor or labor that slows down or stops at different stages.

3. Breech position—This occurs when a baby's feet or buttocks are closer to the pelvis than the head.
4. Fetal distress—This can mean that the baby doesn't seem to be getting enough oxygen, the heart beat is erratic, or something else is wrong.

Hospital C-section rates vary, some hovering around 25 percent, and others at 15 to 17 percent. New York and Massachusetts are two states that have enacted the Maternity Information Act, which requires hospitals in these states to distribute a pamphlet with information about maternity procedures, including C-section rates.

If you really want to avoid a needless cesarean, it's important to find out the C-section rate at the hospital you are considering. In *Unnecessary Cesarean Sections*, the authors provide the C-section rate for hospitals around the country, by state. This makes it easy to identify those hospitals where C-sections are not standard procedure. It's also a good idea to get help from local cesarean-prevention organizations. (See the list of resources at the back of the book.) These organizations keep tabs on hospitals with low cesarean rates, doctors who are less apt to do C-sections, and labor assistants. They are a great resource.

Granted, some C-sections are essential in saving the life of baby and mother. In these birth stories, Sarah Ryan experienced every phase of labor, except the birth. Megan Howard found out that birthing naturally might harm her baby. These two women, under the care of midwives, knew that their C-sections were necessary. Similarly, Kari Garcia Fisher and Jane Gerson faced medical emergencies that were best taken care of by C-section.

On the other hand, it seems that Beth Curry's and Ivy Ratafia's first births did not have to be C-sections. In their stories, you can see how their labors were taken away from them—step by gradual step. One small thing went wrong, and that started the chain reaction of intervention. For Beth Curry, it was being told by a nurse to breathe rapidly. This caused her to hyperventilate and feel faint. At that point, she became a "medical emergency." Ivy Ratafia was handling the contractions well until she was given a drug to help her rest. The drug didn't make her sleepy; it made her feel uneasy and less in touch with her body.

What can be done to make a C-section a better experience? Most women want to have their husbands and/or midwives with them during the operation. It makes them feel less vulnerable. For Megan Howard, having her midwife sit next to her during the operation was a big help. Cynthia held her hand and offered support.

If they are able, women want to see the baby as soon as it's born and to hold it as soon as possible. As Beth Curry and Susan Olman found in their C-sections, if you don't see the baby come out, you might doubt whether the baby is yours. Being able to look at the baby or having it placed on top of you immediately afterward (even if only for a few minutes) enables a mother to make contact with her child.

Note how the women who had C-sections were able to look at the positive side of their experience. If you understand why you have had a C-section and have been part of the decision-making process (and can say, like Megan Howard, "I own this decision"), you will be further along in accepting that this was the way your child had to come into the world.

22

FINDING THE RIGHT CAREGIVER

Your caregiver is the practitioner—obstetrician, family practitioner, or midwife—whom you choose to deliver your baby. Having a good relationship with that person is crucial to your positive birth experience.

In 1993, most women in America (94 percent) gave birth with a physician, whereas only about 5 percent chose to deliver with a midwife. Despite the majority of women choosing physicians, the use of midwives is on the increase. Many women are realizing that there is a big difference between the way physicians and midwives approach labor and delivery.

OBSTETRICIANS

Not all obstetricians are alike. Many believe that childbirth is a medical condition that is best taken care of in the hospital where it can be monitored and controlled. These physicians often approach childbirth from a technical, medical perspective because they have been trained that way. Trained as surgeons, obstetricians generally believe that technology can greatly aid in childbirth. There are certain pressures that also feed the use of technology. One is the concern that mother and baby will survive. Obstetricians also worry about lawsuits. According to a 1990 survey by the American College of Obstetricians and Gynecologists, obstetricians are one of the specialists most likely to be sued, and more than 75 percent have been.

Other physicians take a more holistic approach to childbirth, similar to that of midwives. These doctors usually have low C-section rates, less use of painkillers and epidurals, and a lower episiotomy rate. These doctors are available, but you might have to work to find them. You can contact midwives and ask about their backup doctors. These doctors, because they often work with midwives and understand the midwife philosophy, usually have lower C-section rates than other doctors. You can also contact a local cesarean-prevention organization, such as the International Cesarean Awareness Network. They have lists of physicians with low C-section and intervention rates.

MIDWIVES

The word *midwife* means "with woman." Before the 1800s in the United States, midwives, almost always women, were the primary caregivers during pregnancy and childbirth. But as more women turned to hospitals to have births, they also turned to male professionals, obstetricians, and births involving more technology.

Certified nurse-midwives (CNMs) receive training as nurses and then spend an additional year in a hospital focusing on obstetrics. They practice in hospitals, in birth centers, and in homes. Direct-entry midwives, or lay-midwives, receive on-the-job training and are educated in schools and as apprentices. There is no national standard for their training.

Direct-entry midwives usually practice in private birth centers and in homes.

Midwives have varying legal status across the United States, depending on the state. In some states midwifery is permitted if practiced by an RN or CNM. In California and certain other states, direct-entry midwifery is illegal. When Sarah Ryan gave birth, her midwife could not accompany her to the hospital because not only she did not have hospital privileges, but it was illegal for her to practice there. In New Mexico where lay-midwives are legal, Annette Cantor could have had her midwife accompany her to the hospital if it had been necessary.

Midwives try to offer family-centered care in which the woman is not treated as alone in this experience, according to Kate Scanlan, senior technical adviser for the American College of Nurse-Midwives. The woman is "part of a family and a bigger social context," said Scanlan. "Most women want to be considered individually and don't want to see ten different doctors, or a different caregiver during each visit. That can have an impact on how comfortable she is and on her ability to retain information. There is no reason an obstetrician can't provide these things, but their background is different [from that of midwives]. Obstetrical services are based on the idea that birth is not normal, or that it's subject to complication."

Because of the way midwives' practice is set up, they are able to offer individual care and attention—both during office visits and the birth itself. An office visit with a midwife usually includes time for questions and answers, as well as an exam. Also, midwives usually stay with a woman throughout her labor, instead of just being available during the delivery. Having the support of a midwife means that a woman in labor has a built-in coach—someone to make suggestions about different positions to try, for example. Studies show that, both in this country and others, births with midwives involve less drugs, fewer interventions, and lower C-section rates. In Holland, for example, where midwives are trained as such and don't work under obstetricians, a 1991 study showed lower perinatal mortality rates for midwives compared with obstetricians.

It is not uncommon for your choice of a midwife to be misunderstood by family and friends. This happened to Kari Garcia Fisher when her husband's family from Nicaragua couldn't understand why she would choose a midwife when she could have a doctor. My parents, too, knew more about doctors than midwives and were concerned about my decision to switch to a midwife. They didn't fully understand my choice until after Sam was born and they saw what great shape he was in. Now they have a completely different notion of midwives and what they can do.

QUESTIONS TO ASK YOUR CAREGIVER

Whether you are meeting a caregiver for the first time or are considering using your current doctor, you must ask questions to uncover his or her philosophy about childbirth. It is the answers to these questions that will determine how happy you are and the kind of experience you'll have. You'll want to find a caregiver whose thoughts about childbirth are similar to your own.

Here are some questions to pose to potential caregivers:

Describe a typical birth. Do you require use of IV? Fetal monitoring?

What's the average on-call schedule? What are my chances of being delivered by this doctor or by a partner or other doctor?

How busy is the practice? Is it likely that the caregiver will be delivering other women at the same time?

Do you put any time limits on labor?

What do you do if labor slows down?

How many patients receive painkillers? Which kinds are used?

How many patients receive epidurals? When, during labor, is this usually given?

What positions do you recommend during the pushing phase?

Are forceps ever used? In what circumstances?

Is vacuum extraction ever used? In what circumstances?

Are episiotomies given routinely? Or do you believe in allowing a woman to tear?

What is the C-section rate?

With which anesthesiologists do you work?

If I need a C-section, will you allow my husband to stay with me during the operation?

Do you recommend that I write out a birth plan? Do you and your staff look at them?

You will have a good sense of your practitioner's manner from the way in which your questions are answered. Is the caregiver defensive or evasive? How easy is it to discuss these topics? Trust your instincts. If these questions bring about an uncomfortable discussion or a conversation in which you feel patronized ("Don't worry, I'll take care of everything"), that's a clue that this doctor might not want to hear your thoughts about childbirth—and an indication of the kind of birth offered in the practice. Remember that it's easier to negotiate for what you want during office visits than during labor. If you can find a caregiver whose philosophy about childbirth is similar to your own, you won't have to argue for what you want. Depending on how many different caregivers are available in your area, you might be able to find one whose ideas about birth are similar to your own. "If you have to fight for what you want, you're not where you should be during childbirth," said CNM Carol Bronte.

A word of warning: It isn't always easy to ask a physician these questions. Some doctors don't want to answer them.

(And that's a big clue right there.) Beth Curry took her doctor's nonanswers as agreement and found out later that she had been wrong to make that assumption. My doctor tried to laugh off my concerns about natural childbirth with a know-it-all attitude. She just assumed I trusted her implicitly. I didn't.

Whenever possible, speak to other patients about their experience with a particular caregiver. How someone else is treated is a good indication of how you will be.

Communicating what you want isn't always easy. It's so important, though, that in *Your Baby, Your Way*, Sheila Kitzinger devoted a whole chapter, "Saying What You Want," to the need for the pregnant woman to be assertive. Here's what Kitzinger said about it: "It takes courage to move away from the carefully created image of a woman who always understands, sympathizes, and can put herself in another person's place, to the different image of a decisive, go-getting woman who refuses to take no for an answer, who can state her case with verve, stand her ground, and employ a planned strategy to achieve what is important to her. As women, we have been conditioned not to like ourselves this way. But when you are having a baby, it is really worth it."

The stories here show that getting what you want from your caregiver can mean a world of difference in how you feel about your birth.

It's Never Too Late to Change Caregivers

Both Barbara Cattermole and I changed caregivers late in our pregnancies. Sure, the prospect of being cared for by someone you don't know is daunting. But finding someone whose ideas about childbirth agree with your own makes you feel compatible in no time. In two visits, Barbara Cattermole felt she knew her midwives better than she'd known her doctors after eight months.

In both Barbara's case and my own, our doctors, dismayed that we were dissatisfied and wanted to leave their practices, tried to get us to stay. Barbara and I would have none of it. By that point, we were both so frustrated with our experiences that turning to a midwifery practice (and for Barbara, a birth center) was the only way to go. The morale here is don't be swayed by a practitioner. There are many out there. Find one you really like. It will be worth the effort.

When Rosemary Moore found out that she was having twins, she didn't like her original doctor's response—that she would automatically be put on bedrest and probably have a cesarean. Rosemary knew that she would have to find a caregiver whose philosophy was more in keeping with her own. Susan Olman struggled with a variety of caregivers, often arguing with them about the use of ultrasound, the benefits of going into labor, and the negative effects of a C-section. One of Susan's doctors noted that he was not used to patients like Susan, who cared enough to argue about childbirth.

TRUST, TRUST, TRUST

Many childbirth experts say that the most important aspect of a positive experience is a mother's relationship with her caregiver. If she has a good, trusting relationship, she has everything. If she has confidence in her caregiver, then she can be sure that when decisions are made, they are being made for the right reasons.

"It's a matter of selecting a provider as you would a partner," said Kate Scanlan. "Know what's really important to you about the childbirth experience. If the provider contradicts anything on the list, it's a warning sign. A woman can predict what her experience will be with the statistics of a hospital and doctor."

Both Val Harper and Miriam Block trusted their doctors implicitly. Miriam's trust also extended to her doctor's affiliates. Megan Howard trusted her midwife. For her, this was especially helpful when she had a C-section, and knew her midwife completely backed her decision. Liz Benson's doctor knew that she liked to know all the options available to her. Their conversations—whether during prenatal visits, during the C-section, or, later, during the VBAC—followed suit. For Joanna Allen, trust with her doctor was mutual. Through Joanna's prenatal care, when she often went into dangerously early labor, the doctor knew that Joanna could monitor herself. Conversely, Joanna trusted the decisions her doctor made on her behalf.

THE ROLE OF THE SUPPORT PERSON

Having support during labor is important, so much so that it's mentioned as an alternative to having a painkiller. Having another woman serve as a labor assistant, coach, or *doula* can speed up labor and reduce intervention. As you've seen in these birth stories, a *doula* or coach is a knowledgeable and experienced labor companion hired to provide comfort, support, and encouragement during labor and delivery. In 1991, the *Journal of the American Medical Association* reported a hospital study in which one group of women had a *doula*, and the other didn't. The study found that *doulas* were especially helpful in making childbirth more healthful, safer, and less costly. Pitocin, a drug to induce labor, was used less often, as were epidurals, forceps during delivery, and C-sections.

The role of the support person varies depending on where you give birth. If you are in a hospital, with a doctor, you might want a support person during labor to help you negotiate through hospital procedures. That's what Tim Standing and Miriam Block did when they decided to stay with their doctor's practice. They wanted to make sure they had someone with them who knew the hospital and knew about childbirth. It made their own job in the hospital easier. Tim could concentrate on helping Miriam, instead of dealing with the nurses and doctors they didn't know.

Other women in labor use support people differently. Rosemary Moore had a *doula* as a labor coach, not because she was worried about hospital procedure (she was having twins with midwives in a hospital) but because she wanted the extra assistance. And it helped. Having so much support kept her going. So many people believed in what she was doing that she had to believe it herself.

When Beth Curry's labor coach arrived for her home birth, Beth could tell that the atmosphere at home changed. Everyone relaxed. Katie knew all about labor and delivery, and the responsibility was no longer her husband's and son's. Beth could tell the difference between being helped by her labor coach and by her husband. She believes that women in labor need the support of other women, especially of mothers who have given birth and know what the experience is like.

THE BIRTH PLAN

A birth plan is a written statement about what you would like to have happen when you give birth. It's often written as a list. Barbara Cattermole had a birth plan for her third birth at a birth center. Ann Arscott used one for her water birth, as did Miriam Block for her "planned" natural birth.

Some hospitals have their own birth-plan forms that women are asked to fill out. A 1995 study evaluating birth plans used at two hospitals in Australia found that their use increased women's understanding about the process of labor and the options available to them. Women said the birth plans allowed them to express their needs, enhanced confidence, and improved their communication with hospital staff.

I was not encouraged to write a birth plan, and didn't, although I knew exactly what I wanted. Because we'd spoken about it often, my husband knew my views and agreed with them wholeheartedly. I knew from the orientation to the midwives' practice (at which they presented their philosophy in very certain terms) and from conversations with them afterward that my idea of birth matched theirs. My midwife was going to be with me throughout the labor, and so I didn't expect interference from hospital staff.

Nevertheless, writing a birth plan is helpful in outlining your preferences—both for yourself and for those who will be with you during labor and delivery. Try to find out from other mothers if your caregiver honors birth plans.

To really make sure you have the birth plan you want, make sure you choose a caregiver whose philosophy about birth agrees with your own. And once you have chosen very carefully, put your trust in that person.

❦ 23

DEVELOPING A POSITIVE ATTITUDE

Once you have given some thought to your personal preferences and the options available to you, both in choosing a caregiver and a birth place, you're ready to take the last step in preparation—thinking about the mindset needed for a positive experience.

HOW TO GET IN THE RIGHT FRAME OF MIND

Extricate yourself from the world as we know it. You are having a baby, and you've reached your due date. You feel great physically and mentally. You look wonderful. You are ready and eager for the experience that lies ahead. You aren't worried about what's going to happen because you feel so confident in where you are delivering and with whom. You're ready to go with the flow. It will feel a little like going on a roller coaster, anticipating the swings and high places, but you're ready for that, too. You've been to the room where you'll give birth a thousand times in your mind and know just what it will look like. It's a room with which you're comfortable. You know the people who will be with you. They are loving and kind, and you know exactly what each of them will do for you during labor—a massage, words of support, a hand to hold. You can't wait to see the baby's face. You're ready.

What's wrong with this scenario? There's no worry, no hassle. Nothing unfamiliar, even though all is unfamiliar. What makes this monologue different from the one that might be playing in your head? The difference is that you aren't used to this one. You aren't used to being told that you can do this, that everything is all right. You probably have not grown up hearing over and over again that you can give birth—and give birth well.

Our culture does not reflect the notion that women are equipped to give birth without medical assistance. It does not empower us to believe in our ability to give birth. More likely than not, the TV shows, commercials, and movies that include any kind of childbirth scenes present a stereotype of a medical birth. In a recent TV commercial, a pregnant woman jolts out of bed. "It's time," she says to her husband, and they make their way to the hospital. In TV sit-coms and movies, labor is dramatized as much as it can be to make it as interesting as possible to viewers. Unfortunately, these are the only images we see about childbirth. The laboring woman is in terrible pain, unable to help herself. Or she's in the hospital, lying flat in bed, having things done to her. Women are not usually portrayed laboring at home or shown dealing with their labor. The contractions always seem to come out of the blue. They're a shock. They never come on slow and easy. So is it any wonder that we have to make such a leap when the real thing happens? We are not taught to think that we can handle childbirth.

"If a girl doesn't believe women's bodies are capable of giving birth, she'll grow into a woman who isn't capable," wrote Nancy Wainer Cohen and Lois Estner in *Silent Knife: Cesarean Prevention and Vaginal Birth after Cesarean*. "If a boy integrates messages that birth is dangerous and difficult, he'll grow into a man who has difficulty lending total calm and support to his laboring woman. For both men and women, reeducation is essential."

A friend of mine once confessed that although she had a short labor with her first child, she believed that she ended up with a forceps delivery because she hadn't been "programmed" to think she could give birth. Her mother hadn't had good birthing experiences, and, therefore, the friend thought she couldn't either.

If we don't grow up receiving reinforcing images that we can handle childbirth, we must seek these positive messages elsewhere. Many women do. They find them in the stories of women who have had good experiences—women who faced childbirth as though it was a challenge.

I've heard women refer to childbirth as an adventure. I've heard them express excitement about the idea that another person is about to join them. During a long labor, it's not unusual for women to compare themselves to athletes. Rosemary Moore felt as though she was a long-distance runner, in it for the long haul. Adrienne Rich compared endurance events to childbirth in her book, *Of Woman Born*: "A woman preparing to swim the English Channel, or to climb in high altitudes, is aware that her system will undergo stress, her courage will be tested, and her life may even be in danger; but despite the demands to be expected on her heart, her lungs, her muscular coordination, her nerves, during such an effort, she thinks primarily in terms not of pain but of challenge." Maybe if we can think more in terms of challenge, and less in terms of fear, we will be on our way to better childbirth experiences.

Childbirth educator Barbara Schofield from Brooklyn, New York, has observed that some women come to childbirth class with the "right" attitude. "They have a trust and a belief in their body because that's what their body has taught them over the years. Other women are not as connected to their body's process. They have a vested interest in professionals and in getting that trust from others."

EXPECTATIONS AND REALITY

In the birth stories presented here, several women spoke about what they expected labor to be and how it compared with the real thing. Miriam Block, for example, had seen videotapes of two uncomplicated births and "projected from these." She didn't expect her labor to be as difficult or as long as it was. Rosemary Moore had asked a friend if labor was as painful as "having your arm pulled off." When the friend said yes, Rosemary braced herself for the worst and expected something horrible.

The best advice—from labor coaches, childbirth educators, nurses, and midwives—is to be flexible. Remember that labor is called "labor" for a reason. "People who think they can handle everything sometimes get hit like a ton of bricks," said Carol Bronte. "If you think labor is a breeze, you will be in for a shock. If you expect to work hard, you'll do great. You need to have a healthy respect for it. It hurts."

A word of caution about falling in love with what you're taught in childbirth classes, and so becoming too rigid. Sometimes, couples get so carried away by what they've learned in class that they have a hard time being flexible during labor. It is the Bradley method, which promotes nonmedicated labor, that often gets couples into this trouble. For example, one woman was so enamored of the Bradley method, and wanted natural childbirth so badly, that she fought her doctors when they discovered the baby was in distress. Said Carol Bronte about some couples who take Bradley: "They become fanatic, never-never people. Don't rupture the membranes. Don't take drugs. But I can't have someone whose baby has thick meconium telling me the baby's fine. They become adversarial during labor."

Remember that you can't plan every detail and that your ultimate goal is to deliver a healthy baby safely.

THE PHASES AND EMOTIONS OF LABOR

Many women mention that there is one aspect of the Bradley method that helped them a lot during labor, and that's the Bradley signposts. Because labor is emotional as well as physical, the Bradley method identifies emotional signposts that help a women know how she might feel during each phase of labor. (These signposts are general and refer to a normal labor, not one that is going very fast or is high-risk.) In one of the books often used in Bradley classes, *Natural Childbirth the Bradley Way* by Susan McCutcheon-Rosegg with Peter Rosegg, the signpost chapter is aptly called "The Emotional Map of Labor," acknowledging that labor is both an emotional and a physical experience.

The emotional signposts go something like this:

Phase of Labor	*Emotional Signpost*
During the first part of labor, when the contractions are mild and several minutes apart—	You are excited and happy that labor is starting.
Contractions become more intense—	You are serious about handling the contractions.
Dilation from centimeters 7 to 10—	You feel self-doubt and that you can't go on.

Women like Liz Benson greatly appreciated these signposts. She knew that when the contractions got really hard to handle, she was almost ready to push.

LETTING GO IN LABOR

Some women talk about how they were "out of their heads" or entered a different world during labor. I know that the intensity of labor took me by surprise. Naively, I half-expected, half-hoped that when I reached 10 centimeters, I would get a break and could take a minute to enjoy reaching that goal. But no such thing. Labor doesn't stop at 10 centimeters: it just changes. During the three hours of pushing, I kept dozing on and off. I wasn't aware of everything that was happening to me. I kept saying, "I'm having a reality problem." I felt as though I wasn't really there, and yet I was all there.

What happened to me is similar to what happens to ultra-endurance athletes when they are in the middle of an event. Their minds go elsewhere. Although you won't be able to experience this before it happens, acknowledging that it might could help you prepare for it.

Other women use different tactics to focus during labor. No one plans what they are going to do. It just happens. Said Schofield, "There is a built-in part of the process when you feel like you're not in control. There is a sensory overload as the baby's head comes through or in transition. Most women go through this feeling, when they panic or feel anxious. There is a great value in this adrenalin. It helps to shift us from the last part, when our body is opening, to when we start to push. All this signals into the brain. You can't process it. We need to focus on that."

Some women use a mantra to get through the tough parts of labor. They repeat a word to themselves, finding a pattern of syllables on which to concentrate. One woman I know repeated the word *disassociate*, even though that was the opposite of what she was doing.

When her contractions became intense, Joanna Allen focused on something outside herself. She concentrated on the clock and the monitor, staring at a single object such as a dial.

When you're in the middle of the second phase of labor, time loses meaning. As Rosemary Moore said, three minutes or three hours felt the same to her.

Some women talk about going inside themselves. During Beth Curry's second birth, when labor began to pick up, she focused solely on the contractions, not paying attention to anything else happening around her. Annette Cantor also developed an inward focus and left the outside world behind.

"Some women focus on pain alongside other sensations that are not pain," explained Dr. Heidi Rinehart. "These overwhelming intense sensations can be scary, but they are normal. That's when birth support becomes important. Other things don't do as much for your spirits as human support. There is a struggle to get there, and then there's the beauty from the top."

Once women reach active labor, they are more likely to be overwhelmed than fearful of labor, according to Bronte. "Sometimes you have to talk them down from it. You can say, 'Go with it. Take your time.' If she is running from the chair to the bed, you tell her she can't run away from it. You tell her this is a common feeling, and that she's doing great. You deal with one contraction at a time. You don't think three contractions from now. That works pretty well. I've had women who have not progressed in labor, but not because of outright fear, because of outright control."

YOU DETERMINE YOUR OWN FEELINGS ABOUT CHILDBIRTH

Many couples find that labor is a very intense personal experience. During labor, Tim Standing and Miriam Block discovered aspects of themselves as a couple, and as individuals. Beth

Curry's childbirth experience changed her relationship with herself, her husband, and her son. It also inspired her to rethink her career. Some women find that childbirth is such a charged event that the labor itself, and what happens between husband and wife or between wife and midwife, is a revelation into these personal relationships.

Schofield also acknowledges that childbirth is scary. "It's a healthy thing to approach any big life transition with fear and trepidation. I try to get people to examine what they're worried about and to share that with a partner. It begins to release the charge. It's healthy to face it." Schofield also says that she helps couples recognize the skills they bring to labor; for example, couples already have an established pattern of communication and intimacy that can help during labor.

Couples who are taken aback by their childbirth experience (for example, those who expected to have natural childbirth and ended up with an epidural or cesarean) need to realize that their birth experience is what they make it. "The goal of childbirth is a healthy mother and a healthy baby," says Bronte. "In the continuum of this child's life, the birth experience becomes minor. Get past any negative feelings about what happened during the birth. You have a life to get on with."

Being able to have the childbirth experience you want is powerful and meaningful. The feeling that you can achieve great things extends into all other aspects of your life.

You'll never believe how much you're going to love your baby when it's born. Try to love the "labor" by which he or she comes into this world.

GLOSSARY

Amniocentesis	A test of the amniotic fluid in which the baby floats. It is usually performed between the 16th and 17th week of pregnancy. A needle is placed through the abdomen and into the uterus to take a sample of fluid. The test determines several birth defects and the sex of the baby.
Amniotomy	Artificial rupture of the membranes; when a caregiver "breaks your water."
Anesthesia	Drugs that make the body numb.
Analgesics	Pain-relieving drugs.
Apgar score	A test that determines the alertness and health of a newborn. It looks at skin color, muscle tone, heart rate, level of activity, and respiration rate. The test is usually done at one and five minutes after birth. Scores range from 0 to 10, with a 7 to 10 considered normal.
Braxton-Hicks contractions	Dull, nonlabor uterine contractions.
Breech presentation	Presentation in which the baby's head is up instead of down.

Caput	Swelling that occurs under the baby's scalp.
Certified nurse-midwife	A midwife who is first trained as a nurse and then in midwifery in a hospital setting.
Cervix	The lower part of the uterus.
Dilation	The opening of the cervix.
Doula	A Greek word meaning mothering the mother; a woman who is the caregiver of another woman; can be trained to be with another woman in labor or to administer postpartum care.
Dystocia	Difficult childbirth; usually involves the following circumstances: when labor is slow and doesn't progress very rapidly; or when the baby is too large, the mother's pelvis too small, or the uterus is not contracting efficiently enough to deliver the baby.
Electronic fetal monitoring	Monitoring the baby's heart rate, either by external means (usually a band around the mother's belly) or by an internal monitor attached to the baby's scalp.
Episiotomy	A cut in the perineum to make the vaginal opening bigger for childbirth. It is usually done to prevent the perineum from tearing when the baby is born.

External cephalic version	A manual technique used to turn fetuses from a breech to a head-down position.
Fetal distress	A possible problem with a fetus's health, often meaning lack of oxygen. Variations in electronic fetal monitoring is one way that fetal distress is identified.
Intermittent auscultation	Listening periodically to the fetal heart rate through the mother's abdomen with a stethoscope-type instrument.
IV	Abbreviation for *intravenous*, entering by way of a vein. This allows drugs or fluids to go directly into the bloodstream.
Labor, phases of	
First stage	From the beginning of labor to full (10 centimeters) dilation.
Second stage	Begins with full dilation and ends when the baby is born; the pushing stage.
Third stage	The delivery of the placenta.
Lay midwife	A midwife trained by apprenticeship in a nonhospital setting. Also referred to as a direct-entry midwife.
Meconium	The dark greenish material that accumulates in the baby's bowel during fetal life and is discharged shortly after birth.
Nonstress test	A test of the fetus's heart rate.

Glossary

Oxytocin	The hormone secreted during labor that stimulates contractions.
Perineum	The area between the end of the vagina and the anus.
Pitocin	A synthetic form of oxytocin designed to induce labor.
Preeclampsia	A toxic condition that develops in late pregnancy and that is characterized by such symptoms as high blood pressure, excessive weight gain, and generalized edema.
Transition	The period between the first and second stages of labor, between 8 to 10 centimeters dilated.
Transverse uterine incision	A horizontal incision made in the uterus during a cesarean section.
Ultrasound	A technique used to generate an image by means of sound waves. Also called *sonography*.
Uterine rupture	A tear in a previous scar or in a weak section of the uterus.
VBAC	Vaginal birth after cesarean.
Vertical uterine incision	An up-down incision (also called *classical*) made in the uterus during a cesarean section; no longer used in the United States.

LIST OF RESOURCES

HELPFUL BOOKS

Gabay, Mary, and Sidney M. Wolfe. *Unnecessary Cesarean Sections: Curing A National Epidemic*. Washington, DC: Public Citizen's Health Research Group, 1994.

    This book features a state-by-state list of hospitals that shows their cesarean and VBAC rates.

Goer, Henci. *Obstetric Myths Versus Research Realities*. Westport, CT: Bergin & Garvey Publishers, 1995.

    This book explains how to read and interpret medical literature. It also shows how medical literature can debunk the myths of childbirth. For example, Goer presents studies that show that electronic fetal monitoring does not have a substantial effect on perinatal events. This is a valuable tool for anyone who wants to be well-armed with information in order to get past what doctors might say.

Harrison, Michelle. *A Woman in Residence*. New York, NY: Penguin Books, 1982.

    The subtitle of this book says it all—it's "a doctor's personal and professional battle against an insensitive medical system." It's an inside look at medical care, and what can happen if you are not alert about choosing the right caregiver and hospital.

Kitzinger, Sheila. *Your Baby, Your Way*. New York, NY: Pantheon Books, 1987.
   This book is one of many written by Kitzinger, a noted British childbirth expert. Each of her books is a great resource.

Korte, Diana, and Roberta Scaer. *A Good Birth, A Safe Birth*. Boston, MA: The Harvard Common Press, 1992.
   This book provides a good overview of the medical profession and its take on birth, in order to help readers take control of their own childbirth experience.

McCartney, Marion, and Antonia van der Meer. *The Midwife's Pregnancy and Childbirth Book*. New York, NY: Henry Holt and Company, 1990.
   Although it includes all kinds of information about pregnancy and prenatal care, this book is especially helpful in explaining why women may not want certain procedures in childbirth (for example, painkillers and electronic fetal monitoring). It explains when these interventions may be necessary and also how to avoid them when they are not.

McCutcheon-Rosegg, Susan, with Peter Rosegg. *Natural Childbirth the Bradley Way*. New York, NY: Penguin Books, 1984.
   The Bradley textbook used in many childbirth classes, this book offers easy-to-understand information on what happens inside your body during labor and delivery.

Mitford, Jessica. *The American Way of Birth*. New York, NY: Penguin Books, 1992.
   This book discusses the history of childbirth, from medieval Europe to America today.

Rich, Adrienne. *Of Woman Born*. New York, NY: W.W. Norton & Company, 1986.

Rich takes on the institution of motherhood. This book has several fine chapters on the history of childbirth and on childbirth as it relates to our experience as mothers.

Rothman, Barbara Katz, editor. *The Encyclopedia of Childbearing.* New York, NY: Henry Holt and Company, 1993.
This encyclopedia includes sections written by notable childbirth experts in all areas. It's helpful in answering all kinds of questions about the history and politics of childbirth.

ORGANIZATIONS

Caregivers and Labor Assistants

American College of Nurse-Midwives
818 Connecticut Ave. NW Suite 900
Washington, DC 20006
(202) 728-9860

Doulas of North America
1100 23rd Avenue East
Seattle, Washington 98112
(206) 324-5440

Birth Centers

National Association of Childbearing Centers
3123 Gottschall Road
Perkiomenville, PA 18074
(215) 234-8068

List of Resources

Maternity Center Association
281 Park Avenue South
New York, NY 10010
(212) 777-5000

Home Births, Midwives, and Birth Centers (alternatives to hospital births)

National Association of Parents & Professionals for Safe
Alternatives in Childbirth
Route 1, Box 646
Marble Hill, MO 63764
(573) 238-2010

Cesarean Births and VBACs

C/SEC, Inc.
(Cesareans/Support, Education & Concern)
22 Forest Road
Framingham, MA 01701
(508) 877-8266

International Cesarean Awareness Network (ICAN)
1304 Kingsdale Avenue
Redondo Beach, CA 90278
(310) 542-6400

Childbirth Education Associations
American Academy of Husband-Coached Labor
(Bradley Method)
PO Box 5224
Sherman Oaks, CA 91413
(800) 423-2397

American Society for Psychoprophylaxis in Obstetrics
(Lamaze Method)
1200 19th St. NW Suite 300
Washington, DC 20036
(800) 368-4404

International Childbirth Education Association
PO Box 20048
Minneapolis, MN 55420
(612) 854-8660

Breastfeeding

La Leche League International, Inc.
PO Box 1209
Franklin Park, IL 60131-8209
(800) LA-LECHE

ON-LINE INFORMATION

(Please note that web sites change frequently. This list includes some of the largest and most complete on-line locations.)

The On-Line Birth Center, maintained by Donna Dolezal Zelzer
www.efn.org/~djz
    This is one of the most extensive on-line sites offering information about pregnancy, birth, midwifery, and breastfeeding). From this central address, you'll find links to other childbirth sites of interest on the web.

Another extensive location is www.childbirth.org

Newsgroup:misc.kids.pregnancy is one of the most popular chat sites on the web for pregnancy and childbirth.

The following addresses could include links to other sites:

Obstetric Ultrasound Home Page (includes photos of fetuses)
www.hkstar.com/~joewoo/joewoo2.html

Childbirth Instruction Home Pages
www.bradleybirth.com
www.icea.org
www.lamaze-childbirth.org
www.icea.org

VBAC Home Page
www.childbirth.org/section/VBACindex.html

Home Birth Home Page
http:www.islandnet.com/~browns/homebirth/
homebirth.html

Association of Labor Assistants and Childbirth Educators
www.alace.org

Doulas of North America
http:www.dona.com/index.html

Doula Care Home Page (postpartum)
http:www.webspan.net/~callahan

Lactation Home Page
www.mcs.com/~auerbach/lactation.html

INDEX

Index

Index

Index